NOURISH
The Cancer Care Cookbook

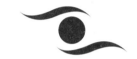

Penny Brohn
Cancer Care

with **Christine Bailey**

dbp

DUNCAN BAIRD PUBLISHERS

LONDON

NOURISH

Penny Brohn Cancer Care
with Christine Bailey

First published in the United Kingdom
and Ireland in 2013 by Duncan Baird Publishers,
an imprint of Watkins Publishing Limited
Sixth Floor
75 Wells Street
London W1T 3QH

A member of Osprey Group

Managing Editor: Grace Cheetham
Editor: Jan Cutler
Managing Designer: Luana Gobbo
Production: Uzma Taj
Commissioned Photography: William Lingwood
Food Stylist: Emily Jonzen
Prop Stylist: Lucy Harvey

A CIP record for this book is available from the
British Library

ISBN: 978-1-84899-076-0

10 9 8 7 6 5 4 3 2 1

Typeset in Adobe Caslon Pro
Colour reproduction by XY Digital
Printed in Italy by L.e.g.o. S.p.a.

Publisher's note The information in this book is not intended as
a substitute for professional medical advice and treatment. If you
have any special dietary requirements or medical conditions or if
you are pregnant or breastfeeding, it is recommended that you
consult a medical professional before following any of the
information or recipes contained in this book. Watkins
Publishing Ltd, or any other persons who have been involved in
working on this publication, cannot accept responsibility for any
errors or omissions, inadvertent or not, that may be found in the
recipes or text, nor for any problems that may arise as a result of
preparing one of these recipes or following the advice contained
in this work.

Notes on the recipes Unless otherwise stated:
• Use medium eggs, fruit and vegetables
• Use organic ingredients, where possible
• Use meat from animals that have been grass fed
• Use organic or free-range eggs
• Use gluten-free, dairy-free and low-salt home-made stock or
  cubes or granules
• Use wild Alaskan salmon
• Do not mix metric and imperial measurements
• 1 tsp = 5ml   1 tbsp = 15ml   1 cup = 250ml

Some recipes also include healthy alternatives. If possible, use
the following ingredients where specified: coconut oil for
cooking; nutritional yeast flakes; and raw cacao powder or cacao
nibs in place of cocoa powder or chocolate.

The food symbols refer to the recipes only, not to any serving
suggestions. Pine nuts have been classed as nuts. Honey,
molasses, xylitol and stevia have been classed as sugars. Check
the manufacturer's labelling, because the ingredients used in
different brands vary, especially for small quantities of
ingredients such as soya and sugar, although manufacturers are
not required to detail minuscule quantities of ingredients.

Acknowledgements Penny Brohn Cancer Care would like to
thank staff: Wendy Burley, BA (Hons), DNTh, MBant, PGCert,
Lead Nutritional Therapist; Dr Catherine Zollman, MRCP,
MRCGP, Fellow in Integrative Medicine, Lead Integrative
Doctor; Dr Eleni Tsiompanou, MD, Diploma in History and
Philosophy of Medicine, MSc in Nutritional Medicine,
Integrative Doctor. With special thanks to funders: The Gerald
Micklem Charitable Trust, The Cyril Corden Trust, The
February Foundation, The Sir Charles Jessel Charitable Trust,
The Coutts Charitable Trust. Thank you also to the nutrition
and services teams and the chefs at Penny Brohn Cancer Care,
who contributed to the work of the cookbook, and to all those
who tested the recipes.

Contents

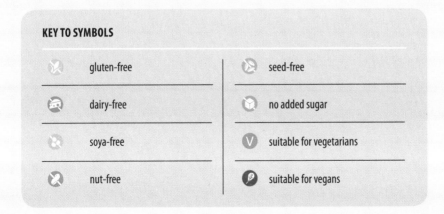

KEY TO SYMBOLS

gluten-free		seed-free	
dairy-free		no added sugar	
soya-free		suitable for vegetarians	
nut-free		suitable for vegans	

Our Whole-Person Approach

Eating well is a simple and powerful way to strengthen your body's natural defences against cancer. We aim to help you enjoy nourishing food and a whole-person lifestyle. Our understanding is based on more than 30 years' experience of helping people to live well with the impact of cancer.

Penny Brohn Cancer Care has supported tens of thousands of people since 1980, as they take this step and make other simple lifestyle changes. Our approach, which has become known as The Bristol Approach, is a powerful combination of physical, emotional, psychological and spiritual support that is designed to help anyone affected by cancer, at any stage of the disease.

Working alongside medical treatment, our philosophy encourages people to build up their own resilience and to harness the power of their body's innate capacity to restore balance and well-being (the technical term for this is homeostasis). We are the leading UK charity working in this field.

When Penny Brohn was diagnosed with cancer in 1979 she asked, "Is there anything that I can do to help increase my chances of staying well?" It set her on the path that led her, and her friend Pat Pilkington, to found the charity that is now known as Penny Brohn Cancer Care. The philosophy was to take a whole-person approach to managing cancer – and this continues to be our aim today.

Nourish is for people affected by cancer, including their family and friends – although much of the information applies to anyone, whatever their age or state of health. It is a source of recipes, inspiration and practical nutritional information that can increase your chances of staying well.

How does a whole-person approach affect cancer cells?

Cancer is a complex group of diseases. There are many different types, with numerous causes. Each cancer type can affect our bodies in a number of ways. In essence, each cancer starts life as a normal cell in which the DNA has been damaged. The damaged cell divides rapidly, multiplying and invading areas of the body where it would not normally be found.

Cancer is often caused by free-radical damage, which creates "oxidative stress" in the body. It uses processes such as angiogenesis (page 13) to grow and spread, and may be encouraged by certain environments in the body, such as inflammation.

The good news is that your body is hard-wired to heal. Your immune system is designed to protect you from all kinds of damage and has specialized white blood cells whose job it is to detect and destroy cancer cells. How a cancer develops depends on the balance between the damaged cells and the ability of your body's immune system to detect and destroy them. Learning how to support your immune system is an essential step towards making your body a less cancer-friendly environment. This is especially important during cancer treatment, which often has the side effect of temporarily reducing immune function.

Your immune system is sensitive to changes in your physical, emotional and psychological states. There may be times when you seem to catch every cold going, especially when you've been under pressure or have been burning the candle at both ends. Now, scientists have proved that white blood cells can be activated or deactivated by chemicals produced in the body; for example, adrenaline and cortisol, which your adrenal glands make when you are stressed, are powerful immune suppressants, whereas endorphins – produced by your body when you exercise – are immune enhancers.

Fortunately, many of the things that keep your immune system working well also make you feel good, so it is a question of listening to your body and finding the right balance for you.

Eating well and exercising regularly, managing your stress and emotions, and connecting to the things and people that really matter in your life are all ways that may help to increase your chances of staying well.

THE FIRST SIMPLE STEPS TOWARDS A WHOLE-PERSON APPROACH

• Eat more whole foods, especially vegetables and fruit, and fewer processed foods.

• Aim to build up to taking some form of exercise for 20 minutes, five times a week.

• Identify any major sources of stress in your life and, if these can't be changed, use regular mindfulness meditation or relaxation to help minimize the effects of the stress on your health.

• Make sure you have support for expressing your emotions when you need to; for example, a cancer nurse specialist, your doctor, through counselling, a support group, friends or family, or by using an online forum or keeping a diary.

• Do at least one small thing every day that lifts your spirits or connects you to the things that matter to you.

Can changing your lifestyle really alter cancer growth?

Researchers who have studied whole-person approaches have found that when people eat more healthily, exercise more regularly and pay attention to managing their stress and emotions, their cancers can sometimes become less active and even shrink in size. Evidence confirms the benefits of such lifestyle changes and how they can increase survival in people with cancer.

These results don't in any way suggest that medical treatments are not needed – this approach can work even more effectively when combined with conventional care – but they do highlight the potential benefits of a whole-person approach for the many millions of people living with a cancer diagnosis in the world today.

You, food and *Nourish*

For many people, improving their diet is the first step towards managing their cancer, and this cookbook will help you to do that. There is more to our approach than the food you eat. The benefit you get from eating well depends on many things;

if you eat meals "on the run", for example, blood flow will be diverted away from your digestive organs so that even if you eat healthily your body may be unable to use the food as well as it could, reducing some of the nutritional benefit. Similarly, if worry about your health is causing lack of sleep or arguments with your family, or if you don't exercise, the overall benefit of the good food you eat may be reduced. What is more, if you're tired, stressed or depressed, you are likely to spend less time cooking and may be more likely to reach for comfort foods instead, which tend to be high in sugar, salt and unhealthy fats – precisely the foods that undermine the body's ability to heal itself.

The intention behind *Nourish* is to help you to adopt healthy eating as a lifestyle. We take you step by step through our approach, explaining at each stage why the food combinations we suggest make a difference to the way your body is able to deal with cancer cells and cancer treatments. In The Link Between Diet & Cancer (page 12) we explain the science behind our approach and what this means for you in practical terms. In How to Eat Well (page 36) there are tips on how to plan, prepare and eat your meals in a relaxed way. There are also suggestions to help you get the most from the food you eat by making sure your digestion is working at its best.

We hope that by reading and using *Nourish* you will be inspired to have fun experimenting with new ideas, new foods and new ways of eating. You'll learn how to increase your resistance to cancer and, by choosing from the many recipes that we've selected, you'll ensure that mealtimes become a daily opportunity to support yourself and live well.

Bon appétit!

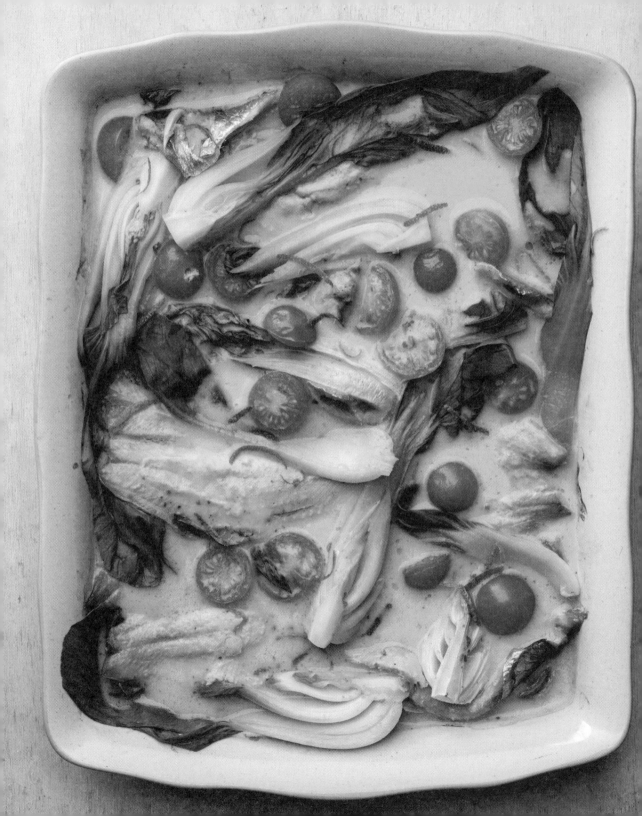

Eat Well, Live Well – Natural Foods & Cancer

In this part we introduce you to the reasoning behind our philosophy at Penny Brohn Cancer Care, and the concepts we adopt for living well with cancer and managing any side effects you may have from treatments. You will find information on foods and nutrition and how it can support your body. We also list the beneficial properties of a variety of foods we recommend you eat often. The daily menu plans at the end of the section will help you decide which meal combinations you may enjoy, using the recipes in the book. Each day's menu focuses on providing a balance of nutrients through a wide range of wholesome foods and flavourings.

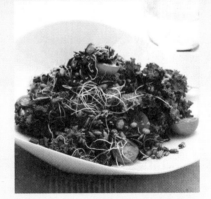

Opposite: Coconut & Lime Baked Sardines (page 80)
Above: Wilted Kale Salad with Toasted Seeds (page 86)

The Link Between Diet & Cancer

Cancer is on the increase, and it is estimated that 50 per cent of people alive today will be diagnosed with the disease in their lifetime. Experts from the World Cancer Research Fund and the American Institute for Cancer Research reviewed the evidence in 2007 and agreed that diet is the single most important factor responsible for this massive rise. It is likely to be responsible for 35 per cent of all cancers – an even greater risk than cigarette smoking. They issued clear guidelines: aim to be slim without being underweight; avoid sugary drinks; eat a variety of healthy whole foods, mainly of plant origin; eat less red and processed meats; and limit alcohol and salt intake.

To understand why diet makes such a difference, it helps to know a little about how cancer develops. Cancer takes advantage of unhealthy environments in the body and uses sophisticated processes to spread. Some of these environments and processes are explained below, as well as how good food can help to protect you.

Why avoiding inflammation is important

Persistent inflammation, swelling or redness, creates an environment that supports cancer at all stages of tumour development, and so foods that help to minimize this are very important. If you include in your diet more omega-3 fatty acids (found in oily fish) but fewer omega-6 essential fatty acids (found in polyunsaturated cooking oils, such as sunflower and vegetable, and in margarines and processed foods), this helps your body to reduce any inflammation. The fibre, vitamins and other antioxidants found in fruit, vegetables and whole grains can also help to reduce inflammation. What is more, recent research shows that omega-3 fatty acids may be able to boost the anti-cancer effect of the breast-cancer drug Tamoxifen.

On the other hand, trans-fats (found in margarines and processed foods) and too many omega-6 fatty acids can encourage inflammation. Not only do they contribute to conditions that favour cancer but they can also contribute to heart disease, atherosclerosis, metabolic syndrome and other chronic conditions.

Beyond this, foods with a high glycaemic index (GI) and glycaemic load (GL) create a pro-inflammatory environment in the body. The glycaemic index and glycaemic load are ways of measuring how quickly the carbohydrates in food are broken down to create glucose in the blood. White bread, white rice (excluding basmati rice), most cereals and foods containing sugar are some of the foods with high GI and GL values. They all make inflammation more likely and/or more pronounced.

Most people enjoy sugar, so it can be hard to accept that it undermines health. Nevertheless, there are several links between sugar, inflammation and cancer growth (see also The Effects of Hormonal Imbalances and Insulin Resistance, page 14), which is why reducing sugar consumption is a major step towards protecting your well-being.

Vitamin D is thought to have a key role in reducing inflammation in the body. Mainly, vitamin D can be made in the body by the daily action of sunlight on the skin, without burning. Vitamin D-rich foods include oily fish, shellfish, egg yolks, mushrooms and butter.

Foods that control the growth of cancer cells

Cancer cells use angiogenesis (the creation of new blood vessels) to supply the oxygen and nutrients they need in order to grow. Angiogenesis is a naturally occurring process in your body, but in a cancerous situation the rate of new blood-vessel formation is abnormally rapid. Scientists have discovered natural food products that help to stop the creation of new blood vessels and are testing them for their potential therapeutic use. By including foods such as shallots, garlic, soya beans, cruciferous vegetables, citrus fruit, spices, green tea and many herbs, you benefit from their anti-angiogenic properties, thereby helping to slow down the creation of the new blood vessels that help cancerous cells to grow.

Slowing down cell division

Cancer cells tend to multiply rapidly, but some foods are able to arrest their growth by interfering with the process of cell division; for example, indole-3-carbinol (I3C) stops cancer cells dividing by locking away an enzyme called elastase. I3C is found in cruciferous vegetables – eating vegetables such as cabbage, cauliflower and broccoli, therefore, slows down the rate at which cancer cells multiply.

Our genes respond to our lifestyle

It is common to believe that our genes determine the risk of developing cancer and that it is coded into our DNA at birth. In fact, only 5–10 per cent of cancers are caused by hereditary factors. Studies from a relatively new branch of biology, called epigenetics, are showing how the genes we inherit are affected by lifestyle, dietary choices and events. This illustrates how genes are not always our destiny and that the lifestyle choices we make can be very powerful in controlling them; a diet rich in folic acid, for example, found in green vegetables, helps to promote healthy epigenetic processes and resists the formation and spread of cancerous cells.

The effects of hormonal imbalances and insulin resistance

Cancer growth can also be stimulated by hormonal imbalances. This is more evident in hormone-sensitive cancers such as breast and prostate cancer. Being overweight or obese increases the risk of these cancers, as well as others including endometrial, colon, pancreatic and kidney.

Obesity also induces insulin resistance. This is where the body no longer tolerates high levels of glucose, causing insulin levels to rise. Insulin works as a growth factor for many cells, especially those in the colon. And, if these cells grow out of control, they can become cancerous. In advanced stages of cancer, insulin resistance contributes to weight loss and feeling weak.

Being a healthy weight is an important step towards protecting yourself from hormone-sensitive cancers, insulin resistance and other chronic diseases.

The damaging effects of stresses on the body

The production of free radicals is a normal chemical reaction in the body; however, we live in a world that promotes the over-production of free radicals: smoking and drinking alcohol, as well as environmental pollution and stress, are just some of the triggers that prompt their formation. When the body is in contact with too many free radicals, it is unable to limit the cell damage they cause, and this accumulates over time. The result is known as oxidative stress, which drives cancer initiation and development. More recent studies suggest that cancer cells may also deliberately create oxidative stress around them to destroy the normal cells and steal their nutrients for their own use.

Antioxidants are chemicals that "mop up" free radicals and reduce their damaging effects. The damage of free radicals in the body can be limited by including foods that are rich in antioxidants, such as vitamins C and E, and the minerals selenium and zinc. Plant foods are your first choice for these nutrients: vegetables, fruit, seeds and nuts. Zinc and selenium are also found in meat and seafood.

Our Approach to Healthy Eating

At the core of the Penny Brohn Cancer Care approach to healthy eating is the belief that foods in their most natural state are the best for you. A whole-food diet based on fresh, unprocessed foods will keep you the healthiest you can be. We recommend a diet based primarily on plant foods, vegetables and fruit, whole grains, pulses, nuts, seeds, herbs and spices. We also recommend some animal products alongside the plant foods, but in a smaller amount.

Organic or not organic?

If you can, choose organically produced foods, particularly animal products. Two good reasons to eat organic are that these foods have lower levels of potentially harmful residues and, according to scientific research, they may have higher levels of beneficial nutrients. Organic foods tend to be relatively more expensive and not so widely available, so you may want to combine organic and non-organic foods in each meal. The most important thing is to eat a wide variety of whole foods.

Food basics in a nutshell

The principles of a cancer-preventative diet are summed up by balance, variety, colour and moderation. Eat a good balance of the different food groups and vary the foods you eat from within those groups – the colour of your food is a good indication of its nutritional value. The more colour variety the more nutrient value.

Choosing what to put on your plate

It's possible that your plate may look quite different from what you have been used to. A large portion of your healthy-eating plate should be made up of vegetables and it will include some other plant foods (fruit, whole grains, pulses, nuts and seeds) too. There will be some protein, either in the form of animal products or pulses. You need protein to build and maintain every cell in your body, and protein in your food

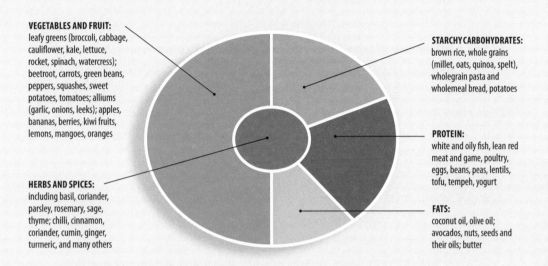

VEGETABLES AND FRUIT:
leafy greens (broccoli, cabbage, cauliflower, kale, lettuce, rocket, spinach, watercress); beetroot, carrots, green beans, peppers, squashes, sweet potatoes, tomatoes; alliums (garlic, onions, leeks); apples, bananas, berries, kiwi fruits, lemons, mangoes, oranges

STARCHY CARBOHYDRATES:
brown rice, whole grains (millet, oats, quinoa, spelt), wholegrain pasta and wholemeal bread, potatoes

PROTEIN:
white and oily fish, lean red meat and game, poultry, eggs, beans, peas, lentils, tofu, tempeh, yogurt

HERBS AND SPICES:
including basil, coriander, parsley, rosemary, sage, thyme; chilli, cinnamon, coriander, cumin, ginger, turmeric, and many others

FATS:
coconut oil, olive oil; avocados, nuts, seeds and their oils; butter

also helps to regulate the release of sugar into your bloodstream. You also need to eat healthy fats, so they should be included on the plate too, in the form of vegetable oils, nuts and seeds, or butter. And finally, if you add some herbs and spices to your plate, you'll boost the flavour of your food and benefit from their powerful health-enhancing properties.

There can be treats too

Follow the healthy-eating guidelines outlined here 90 per cent of the time and the odd treat won't hurt. Most people find that after eating healthy foods for a while, their tastes change, and they prefer wholesome foods. You may find that your old idea of a food treat will no longer appeal in the same way.

You are in control

The simple and general guidelines in the following pages are there to help you assess your own dietary intake and judge whether you need to increase the amount you eat of some types of food and reduce others. Certain foods may be more important on some occasions, whereas others will be more appealing at other times, and you may need to adapt your meals to maintain a good balance.

Foods to eat on a daily basis

Plan to eat the following foods daily and include a wide variety of those listed in the Power of Food chart on pages 24–9.

VEGETABLES AND FRUIT   Various scientific studies have shown that vegetables and fruit can help protect against cancer. They also contain compounds that support health in general, including fibre, vitamins, minerals and phyto (plant) nutrients.

We recommend eight portions of fresh vegetables and two to three portions of fruit every day. Choose a variety of vegetables and fruit in an array of colours, to ensure that you get the full range of important phytonutrients. A simple way to estimate a portion size is to work out the amount of a vegetable or fruit that would fit into your cupped hand.

PROTEIN FOODS   One of the vital roles protein plays in your diet is in helping your body to repair itself. Cells can be damaged by disease, injury, surgery and even treatment, so sufficient protein from the diet is essential. Your body also needs protein to maintain a healthy immune system and to prevent infection.

We recommend some protein at each meal. On average, we would recommend animal products five to six times a week – eggs or a palm-sized portion of meat, poultry or fish. Animal products are good sources of protein and those we particularly recommend are white meat, lean red meat and game, fish and eggs. Ideally, use a variety of animal and vegetable proteins, as they have different properties. If you choose a vegetarian diet, make sure that you regularly eat sources of plant protein – pulses, nuts and seeds – and high-protein grains such as quinoa.

PULSES Also known as legumes, pulses include beans, lentils and peas. They have a relatively high protein content compared to other plant foods, and are also good sources of fibre, vitamins, minerals and phytonutrients, including phytoestrogens.

We recommend a variety of well-cooked or sprouted pulses – sprouting enhances the nutritional benefits. Minimize beans if your digestive system is delicate.

WHOLE GRAINS Grains that are unrefined – whole grains – contain fibre, B vitamins, vitamin E, and a range of minerals and essential fats.

We recommend a variety of whole grains including quinoa, millet, barley, buckwheat and rye as well as spelt (lower in gluten than wheat), wheat, rice and oats. If you are not eating animal products, combine grains with pulses.

HEALTHY FATS Your body requires fats to absorb some nutrients, such as the fat-soluble vitamins and minerals. They also assist brain function and improve insulin resistance. Healthy fats include oils from olives, coconuts, nuts and seeds (ideally cold pressed, because heavy processing damages fats), as well as green leafy vegetables. Animal products also contain healthy fats. Oily fish is a good source of the omega-3 fats.

We recommend both unsaturated and saturated fats, although saturated fats found in meat and high-fat dairy products should play less of a role in the diet than the unsaturated fats found in vegetables, nuts, seeds and oily fish. As omega-3 is often deficient in the average Western diet, aim to eat omega-3-rich foods daily: flaxseed (also called linseed), walnuts, hemp seeds and their oils, oily fish, meat from grass-fed animals and free-range eggs.

Oils can become damaged when heated at high temperatures, and should only be heated to a minimal extent. Saturated fats (such as coconut and animal fats) and monounsaturated fats (such as olive oil) are more stable on heating.

Although butter is a saturated fat, it is far less processed than any type of margarine or low-fat spread and, in moderation, can play a part in a healthy diet.

HERBS AND SPICES Natural flavourings in the form of herbs and spices are a rich source of phytonutrients with powerful health-enhancing properties, including antioxidants and anti-inflammatory capabilities.

We recommend using a variety of herbs and spices on a daily basis. Examples include garlic, ginger, chilli, turmeric, rosemary, mint and thyme. Use fresh or dried in salads, cooked dishes and as teas.

Foods to eat in moderate amounts

RED MEAT Important nutrients including B vitamins and minerals (especially iron) are found in red meat. There is evidence that too much red meat can increase the risk of certain cancers, but there is no health risk associated with eating a moderate amount of unprocessed red meat.

We recommend only eating small portions of red meat – approximately the amount that would fit into the palm of your hand. Choose organic or grass-fed meat, if you can, as the nutrient quality is much higher.

DAIRY PRODUCTS Containing a range of vitamins and minerals, dairy products are a good source of protein and healthy fats. Nevertheless, some researchers have questioned whether they are suitable for people with cancer, especially hormone-sensitive cancers. The research shows dairy to be a risk factor in prostate cancer, although there has been little research examining the effects of dairy produce on the health of cancer survivors. Some people find that, after anti-cancer treatment, dairy foods upset their digestion.

We recommend, for people with prostate cancer and those who find milk products difficult to digest, that you keep the amount of dairy products you eat to a minimum. For others, organic and full-fat yogurt and butter can be used, with minimal amounts of milk and cheese. You may find goat's or sheep's products easier to digest.

SOYA PRODUCTS Foods made with soya beans are an important part of traditional Asian diets (for example, in the form of tofu, miso or tempeh) but they are a relatively new addition to the Western diet. Like some other plant foods, they contain phytoestrogens; however, soya also contains less favourable compounds, often termed "anti-nutrients", that can interfere with nutrient absorption.

We recommend that if you eat soya, choose organic types such as tofu, miso, tempeh and natto, which tend to have lower levels of these anti-nutrients.

Foods to eat in minimal amounts

These foods have little or no health benefits and are best eaten rarely or avoided.

REFINED GRAINS AND SUGARS Products made with refined grains, such as white flour and white rice, lose a lot of their natural nutritional value, including fibre, in the refining process. Eating these refined carbohydrates leads to a rapid rise in blood sugar and encourages unhealthy changes in your body.

We recommend avoiding refined grains and sugary foods as much as possible. Vegetables and fresh or dried fruit are full of natural sweetness and can be used to make healthy puddings, cakes and biscuits.

UNHEALTHY/DAMAGED FATS Fats that have been damaged due to heavy processing are particularly bad for you. Trans-fats are an example. These are mainly found in partially hydrogenated vegetable oils, which are used in commercial crisps, mayonnaise, cakes, biscuits, pastries and deep-fried foods.

We recommend avoiding processed, fatty foods. Instead, prepare cakes, biscuits and pastry products at home using butter or oils such as olive and coconut. Don't heat oils to high temperatures during cooking, as this can cause oxidation and damage the fats, although coconut and rapeseed oils are more stable at higher temperatures.

PROCESSED MEATS There is evidence to suggest that a high intake of processed meats increases the risk of developing some cancers. Processed meats include heavily processed burgers and sausages, salami, bacon and other smoked or cured meats.

We recommend minimizing the amount of processed meat you eat. If you have it occasionally, choose organic products if possible.

BARBECUED, GRILLED AND GRIDDLED FOODS There is evidence that eating lots of barbecued, grilled or griddled foods may increase the risk of certain cancers; however, there is no harm in having these occasionally.

We recommend that when you cook foods in these ways, in particular meat, don't allow them to come into direct contact with a naked flame and try not to allow them to over-brown or burn.

Salt

If processed food forms a large part of your diet, you will most likely be eating too much salt, which can upset the delicate balance of minerals in the body. Whole foods and fresh, unprocessed foods are naturally low in salt. You can use a little good-quality rock or sea salt in cooking to enhance flavour. Also use herbs, spices, garlic, onions, dried mushrooms, dried tomatoes and lemon juice to further enhance flavour. Seaweed can also add flavour and is a valuable source of iodine, which is often deficient in the modern diet.

Water

Drinking enough water to stay well hydrated is an important part of your healthy-eating plan. The best way to do this is to drink regularly throughout the day. An average adult needs between 1.5 litres/52fl oz/6 cups and 2 litres/70fl oz/8 cups of fluid every day. If you are very physically active or the weather is hot, you may want more. Water, herbal teas and fresh vegetable juices can count towards your fluid intake, but keep fruit juices, sugary drinks, caffeinated drinks and alcohol to a minimum.

Moving forward

Dietary needs can change with time as your health, lifestyle and moods alter. Some foods may be particularly appealing at one time but less appealing at another. Using the recipes and information in this book you can choose healthy options that you can be sure will satisfy you, give you pleasure and support your body.

FOODS TO EAT REGULARLY, ON A DAILY BASIS	FOODS TO EAT IN MODERATE AMOUNTS	FOODS TO EAT IN MINIMAL AMOUNTS
Vegetables and fruit	Red meat	Refined grains and sugars
Protein foods	Dairy products	Unhealthy/damaged fats
Pulses	Soya products	Processed meats/foods
Whole grains		Over-browned, burned and barbecued foods
Healthy fats		Salt
Herbs and spices		
DRINKS		
Water	Coffee	Alcohol

The Power of Food – Where to Find the Nutrients You Need

Many of the natural compounds in whole foods have been shown to discourage cancer growth. Combining them in a meal helps to increase their beneficial properties.

Whether you are undergoing cancer treatment, you are in recovery or wanting to prevent the onset or recurrence of cancer, eating nutrient-rich food is a crucial part of your programme. The following charts give examples of nutrient-rich foods, the compounds within them and some possible health benefits.

FOODS	SOME OF THE NATURAL COMPOUNDS	POSSIBLE BENEFITS
Allium vegetables: chives, garlic, leeks, onions, spring onions	Allicin, alliin and the enzyme allinase. Diallyl sulphide and S-allyl cysteine. The flavonoid quercetin	May restrict the growth of cancer cells/tumours and be protective against stomach, gastric and colon cancers. May inhibit breast, liver and colon cancer. May help to reduce the side effects of radiotherapy. Potent antioxidant and anti-microbial. Quercetin is an antioxidant and may protect against hormone cancers. Immune supportive properties
Citrus fruits: grapefruit lemons, limes, oranges; and celery	Bioflavonoids such as ellagic acid, hesperidin, rutin. Limonoids, vitamin C	Antioxidant and anti-inflammatory. They support the immune system and inhibit tumour growth

FOODS	SOME OF THE NATURAL COMPOUNDS	POSSIBLE BENEFITS
Cruciferous and green vegetables: broccoli, Brussels sprouts, cabbage, cauliflower, horseradish, kale, mustard greens, radish, spinach, wasabi, watercress	Carotenoids, indole-3-carbinol, sulphorophane, vitamins C, E and K	Disrupt tumour formation and growth. Promote cancer cell death. Antioxidant and anti-inflammatory
Mushrooms: button, cordyceps, enoki, maitake, reishi, shiitake	Lentian, polysaccharides	Shiitake mushrooms contain 1:3 betaglucan polysaccharides shown to support immunity and destroy cancer cells. Reishi, cordyceps, and maitake encourage the immune system to identify and destroy cancer cells
Orange/yellow vegetables and fruit: apricots, carrots, mangoes, peppers, pumpkins, squashes, sweet potatoes, watermelon	Carotenoids, particularly beta-carotene, lutein, lycopene	An immune-enhancing effect. They have been shown to inhibit cancer cell formation and are potent antioxidants. Some studies have shown beta-carotene supplements can reduce cancer risk by 40 per cent (however, smokers should not supplement with synthetic beta-carotene)
Red vegetables and fruit: acai berries, aubergine, beetroot, blueberries, cherries, cranberries, figs, grapes, pomegranate, raspberries, red cabbage, red plums, strawberries	Anthocyanins, ellagic acid, flavonoids, oligomeric proanthocyanidins, resveratrol	Protect against DNA damage. Reduce the rate of cancer cell growth and cause cancer cell death. They have anti-oestrogen activity, are anti-inflammatory and support immune activity. Many of these compounds have been shown to help prevent breast and prostate cancers

FOODS	SOME OF THE NATURAL COMPOUNDS	POSSIBLE BENEFITS
Tomatoes	Carotenoids, lycopene, vitamin C	Inhibit tumour formation and carcinogenic activity. Harvard Medical School found that eating 10 servings a week could reduce prostate cancer risk by 40 per cent. Fat helps the absorption of lycopene
Beans and pulses	Fibre, isoflavones, phytoestrogens	Inhibit tumour formation. May protect against certain hormonal cancers, such as breast and prostate. Reduce the risk of atherosclerosis, heart disease and osteoporosis
Oily fish: anchovies, mackerel, pilchards, salmon, sardines, trout	Omega-3 fats, vitamin D	Anti-carcinogenic and anti-inflammatory. Regulates the immune system. Slows the growth of tumours and prevents their spread. Effective against hormone-dependent cancers. Avoid eating larger fish such as shark, swordfish, marlin and tuna
Organ meat, especially kidneys and liver	B vitamins, iron, selenium, vitamin D	Increases energy and circulation of oxygen. Antioxidant. Selenium may protect against certain cancers such as breast and prostate cancer
Soya	Genistein, isoflavones, excellent source of complete protein to replace meat	Tissue repair. Can help to balance hormones. Ideally use the whole food product to supply isoflavones rather than an isolated supplement. Choose organic, non-GM soya, preferably fermented

FOODS	SOME OF THE NATURAL COMPOUNDS	POSSIBLE BENEFITS
Apple cider vinegar	Malic acid, pectin, potassium	Supports digestive health and secretion of digestive enzymes. Lowers glycaemic index/load of meals
Butter, ghee	Butyric acid, conjugated linoleic acid (CLA), vitamins A and D	Improve intestinal health. CLA is shown to suppress cancer cells
Coconut: flesh, oil, water and milk	Caprylic acid, lauric acid, medium chain triglycerides	Anti-microbial and anti-cancer properties. Easy to digest
Fermented foods: e.g. live yogurt, miso, sauerkraut	Healthy bacteria (probiotics)	Support digestion, immune function and intestinal health
Flaxseed (linseed) and its oil, nuts, seeds, whole grains	Lignans, magnesium, phytosterols	Modulate oestrogen activity and enhance immune function. Antioxidant activity, anti-bacterial, anti-viral and anti-fungal
Olive oil and avocado oil	Oleic acid, omega-9 fatty acids	Support blood sugar levels. Antioxidant, free-radical scavenger
Sea vegetables: arame, dulse, kelp, kombu, wakame	Fucoidan, iodine	Fucoidans are starch-like (polysaccharide) molecules with anti-inflammatory and anti-viral properties. They are immune enhancing and may reduce the risk of breast cancer. Iodine assists thyroid function and improves metabolism
Tea (matcha, white, green, black), dark chocolate	Polyphenols, e.g. catechins, including epigallocatechin gallate (EGCG)	Antioxidant, anti-inflammatory and anti-angiogenic. Modulate hormone activity and support immune function

HERBS AND SPICES	SOME OF THE NATURAL COMPOUNDS	POSSIBLE BENEFITS
Basil, mint, oregano, rosemary, thyme	Essential oils of the tarpene family	Reduce the spread of cancer cells by blocking enzymes needed to invade other tissue
Coriander	Leaves, essential oils in seeds	A digestive aid. Anti-inflammatory and anti-microbial
Fennel	Coumarin compounds, such as anethole	Reduces inflammation by influencing cell signalling
Parsley	Carotenes, chlorophyll, folic acid, iron, vitamin C	Inhibits the cancer-causing properties of fried foods. A nerve stimulant, useful in energy drinks
Peppermint	Perillyl alcohol, also contains rosmarinic acid	Inhibits the growth of tumours and is a powerful antioxidant
Sage	Flavonoids, rosmarinic acid	Has blood-sugar lowering effects. Anti-microbial and anti-fungal
Chillies	Capsaicin	Anti-microbial. May be particularly effective against certain types of skin cancer
Cinnamon	Essential oils from the bark, e.g. cinnamyl acetate	Helps to balance blood sugar, helps insomnia and optimizes circulation
Cloves	Beta-caryophyllene, eugenol	May prevent digestive-tract cancers. Offers protection from environmental pollution. Used in the treatment of joint inflammation. A mild anaesthetic

HERBS AND SPICES	SOME OF THE NATURAL COMPOUNDS	POSSIBLE BENEFITS
Ginger	Gingerols	Anti-inflammatory, stimulates digestion and soothes the intestinal tract. Promotes circulation
Saffron	Carotenoids, dimethylcrocetin, safranal	Immune-boosting anti-carcinogenic, antioxidant and antidepressant
Turmeric	Curcumin is the main active ingredient in this curry spice	Antioxidant activity and anti-inflammatory, stimulates cancer cell death (apoptosis)

This is just a selection of whole foods and their benefits, and it shows how many contain natural health-giving properties. Don't feel that it is essential to eat specific foods because of their healthy properties, if they don't appeal to you. Always be guided by your taste, and include your favourite foods as well as those ones above that you prefer. Just as we adopt a whole-person approach to our well-being, we should also adopt a synergistic approach to food and meals by combining different foods in one meal or snack.

When planning meals, eat a variety of whole foods in combination, and avoid concentrating on one particular food or compound because of its specific benefit. Choose a food rather than a supplement; enjoy a curry flavoured with turmeric and made with meat, poultry or a vegetarian protein, plus vegetables, rather than taking a turmeric supplement. You will benefit from the anti-inflammatory properties of the curcumin as well as the anti-inflammatory and antioxidant benefits from the healthy fats you cook with, the other curry spices and the foods you have included.

Managing Treatment & Side Effects

What you eat during your cancer treatment really matters, because it helps to keep you strong and can also help you to deal with any problems caused by the treatment. This chapter looks at some of the side effects you can expect from treatment and explains what and how to eat to help you feel better.

Our healthy-eating approach can form the basis of anything you do before, during and after treatment; however, there may be times when you need to adapt our guidelines. Your body, your illness and your circumstances are unique, so use this information accordingly. You may also want to talk to a specialist to receive personalized advice.

Fatigue

Feeling tired is the most common symptom people with cancer experience during and after treatment. Use food to obtain the energy and nutrients that you need.

• Be prepared. Do your shopping online. Cook when you are not tired. Make larger quantities of food and freeze some of it for other days.

• Have nutritious, home-made soups, as they are easy to digest and do not contain energy-depleting additives present in shop-bought foods.

• Drink plenty of fluids, because dehydration depletes energy. Try the juices described in this book. Have a chocolate drink, using your choice of milk or milk substitute. Dark chocolate has a remarkable effect on energy levels. It can also lift your mood.

• Have healthy, nutritious snacks: fresh fruit with nuts or seeds, dried fruit (figs, dates and apricots), dark chocolate, boiled eggs, yogurt, chicken liver or sardine pâté. Your body is better able to digest snacks and small meals than one large meal.

• Aim to be a healthy weight.

Loss of appetite and nausea

A loss of appetite is a complex symptom. It can be caused by treatment or by the cancer itself. Changes to your sense of taste and smell, experiencing a dry mouth, nausea, diarrhoea, constipation, slower digestion of your food, fatigue, low mood or depression, anxiety, pain, breathlessness and infection may all cause you to lose your appetite. Ask for help from your medical team to address what can be treated.

• Try different foods and find what you enjoy most. Sometimes eating smaller meals more frequently can help.

• Always go for the healthier choices. Avoid foods that are difficult to digest, such as deep-fried foods.

• Sometimes gentle foods, such as porridge, are the easiest to eat when you are not hungry or you feel sick. Porridge is quick and easy to make, and has calories to sustain you, as well as antioxidants and fibre. Add some ground seeds and nuts, banana, honey, cinnamon and berries, poached fruit or plums.

• Avoid strong smells, as these may trigger nausea. When you are nauseous, drink plenty of water, mild vegetable juices and herb teas (such as peppermint, as it helps digestion and therefore avoids the side effect of nausea). Ginger may also help to reduce your sickness, so use it in teas and food.

• To improve your appetite, have a walk in the fresh air before you eat.

Changes in taste and smell

Some chemotherapy drugs, as well as certain antibiotics, painkillers and steroids, can make food taste salty, bitter or metallic. Radiotherapy to the head and neck region can damage the taste buds and alter your sense of smell or change taste.

• Avoid red meats, which can have a particularly metallic taste.

• Flavour foods with herbs, spices and lemon juice.

• You may find cold foods more appealing than hot foods.

Difficulty swallowing, oral thrush and mouth ulcers

Swallowing problems and mouth ulcers can be a result of chemotherapy or radiation to the neck or chest area. You may be susceptible to infections, such as oral thrush, which can make swallowing painful, because the cancer and/or its treatment suppresses your immune system.

- If possible, consume fresh vegetable juices to boost your nutrient intake. Cabbage juice is soothing to the throat and the rest of the digestive tract. Mix it with other vegetables and fruit to enhance the flavour.
- Consume softer healthy foods such as bananas, mashed root vegetables (such as sweet potato, parsnip, swede, carrot), rice pudding, home-made soups and casseroles, and cooked fruits. Braise tougher foods such as meat, to tenderize them, and mix them with softer foods to make them easier to eat. You could try blending them, if necessary.
- Take a sip of water (or vegetable juice) between each bite of food, so that the liquid can help to wash the food down between mouthfuls.
- Use a straw if necessary for liquids and blended foods.
- Avoid salty, spicy or acidic foods to prevent further irritation to the mouth.
- Consume as many immune-supporting foods as possible, particularly vegetables and fruit, onions and garlic, shiitake mushrooms, herbs and spices.

Digestive problems: bloating and flatulence, or slower digestion of food

Cancer, its treatment, and even dietary changes (such as rapidly switching to a raw or whole-food diet) can all cause digestive problems. Some people who have had surgery, radiotherapy and/or certain types of chemotherapy, become unable to digest fats, carbohydrates (such as lactose found in dairy products) and proteins (for example, gluten found in wheat and other grains). This may be temporary or permanent. When it happens, it causes abdominal cramps, bloating and flatulence. If raw foods or pulses are new to your diet, introduce them gradually.

It is important to discuss any concerns with a professional, such as a doctor or nutritionally trained practitioner.

Diarrhoea

Treatment, or the cancer itself, can cause diarrhoea, and it may also be the result of stress, food intolerances, or a viral or bacterial infection. If the diarrhoea is severe and prolonged (longer than 2 days), seek help from your doctor.

• Drink plenty of fluids to replace those lost.

• Avoid all dairy products, as the lactose in milk can make diarrhoea worse.

• Avoid hot or very cold drinks.

• Avoid caffeine.

• Avoid greasy and/or heavily spiced foods.

• You may need to reduce your intake of high-fibre foods, but only until the diarrhoea improves. In this case, avoid pulses, whole grains (use white flour, pasta and rice in the short term instead), and raw vegetables and fruit (try peeled, cooked vegetables and fruit instead).

• The insoluble fibre and pectin in apples helps bowel regularity, and may relieve both constipation and diarrhoea.

Constipation

Like diarrhoea, constipation may be due to the cancer itself or its treatment. It may also be caused by poor diet lacking in sufficient fibre, low fluid intake and/or decreased physical activity and weakness.

• Drink plenty of fluids; warm drinks, such as herb teas can be particularly helpful.

• Eat more high-fibre foods, such as whole grains, vegetables and fruit (especially oranges and apples).

• Eat dried fruit, especially prunes and figs, to help keep the bowels moving.

• Gentle exercise may be of benefit.

• Massaging the tummy gently may help to ease blockages.

• Eat slowly and chew well to help digestion.

Maintaining a Healthy Weight

Until recently, people were advised to eat whatever they wanted during cancer treatment to avoid losing weight. Modern knowledge challenges this and stresses the importance of eating a balanced, nutritious diet to maintain a healthy weight.

Weight gain

When you have cancer, you can put on excessive weight for a number of reasons:

• You have certain types of cancer, such as breast, prostate, endometrial, ovarian, colorectal and brain cancer, in which hormonal changes and treatment can encourage weight gain.

• You are taking certain medications, such as steroids and hormonal treatments. Contrary to expectation, many people can also put on excess weight during chemotherapy as well as other treatments.

• You are feeling tired or stressed. You may then turn to eating comfort foods.

• You don't take enough physical activity because of fatigue, discomfort, low mood or habit, or for other reasons.

• You find it hard to change unhealthy eating habits, especially at times of crisis.

To help you achieve a healthy weight, follow the principles set out in this book. Research has shown that a plant-based diet may encourage weight loss in those who are overweight, particularly if combined with regular physical activity.

Maintain a reasonable level of physical activity, without overdoing it. Physical activity, such as walking, will help you to deal with fatigue as well as burning calories and lifting your mood. When exercising aim to lift your spirits as well as increasing your energy. Use meditation, visualization, or relaxation to support yourself and maintain your resolve.

Another useful way to help avoid weight gain is to eat mindfully. Research shows that when we eat slowly and chew well, we feel full quicker and therefore eat less. Remember, though, that each one of us is different. How we deal with weight gain will depend on our circumstances, and these may also change and influence our resolve to do what is best for us. Small changes in eating patterns can make a big difference after a while. If you have a setback it is always worth trying again.

Weight loss

People with cancer can lose weight for many reasons: as a direct effect of the tumour or following cancer treatment (surgery, chemotherapy, radiotherapy). Cancer is a complicated disease and the disease processes that it uses for its survival can sometimes lead to weight loss, often accompanied by a loss of appetite. In certain types of cancer, including lung and pancreatic cancer, this is more common.

If you are losing weight, you may need to eat extra calories, proteins, healthy fats and other nutrients. Healthy, calorie-rich foods include nuts and seeds, dried fruit (figs, dates and prunes), oily fish, avocados, dark chocolate, nut and seed butters, coconut milk and full-fat yogurt. Try our Blueberry Avocado Build-Up Shake, for example. Don't be tempted to fill yourself up with unhealthy fats or sugar.

It may also help you if you follow an anti-inflammatory diet and lifestyle to reduce inflammation, which is linked to cancer growth:

- Eat foods that have anti-inflammatory properties (fruit and vegetables, whole grains, pulses, fish, olive oil and herbs) – see The Power of Food, page 24.
- Avoid foods that lead to inflammation (oils high in omega-6 fatty acids, foods containing trans-fats, commercially fried foods – see page 12).
- As well as eating healthily, take regular exercise, because it inhibits the production of compounds, such as some prostaglandins, which contribute to inflammation.
- Have some exposure to sunshine to create adequate vitamin D: 15 minutes a day without sunscreen, but avoid burning. Adequate vitamin D is essential for immune system functioning and is very commonly deficient in cancer patients.
- Consider taking omega-3 supplements. A diet rich in omega-3 fatty acids has been shown to help people with weight loss in the advanced stages of cancer.

How to Eat Well

It takes just a moment to make the decision to improve your diet, but making those improvements actually happen is a daily process – albeit an exciting one – of discovering new foods, new recipes and new eating routines. This section offers some practical hints and tips on how to make those changes.

Moving on, step by step

- Too many changes at once can be overwhelming and stressful, both physically and emotionally. Do things at a gradual pace that suits you. Even small changes can bring positive benefits that will help to keep you motivated.
- Take time to restock your cupboards and fridge with whole foods.
- Get support. If you have friends or family offering to help, ask them to prepare a meal for you, perhaps something that you can freeze to eat at a later date. Many of the recipes in this book can be frozen or will keep for a few days in the fridge.
- Get advice. Talk to people who are familiar with healthy cooking and ask them for their tips, tricks and ideas.
- Buy standby foods for off-days. A selection of healthy frozen foods is a useful option for days when cooking is too much. Tinned products (such as pulses, tomatoes, fish) and nut and seed butters are also handy to have readily available, but choose those without added sugar or salt. If you always have nuts and fruit at home, you can easily prepare a smoothie.
- Grow your own. Consider growing some herbs in pots, or even planting a small vegetable plot. Freshly picked food, direct from your garden, will be bursting with goodness. Plus, there's the satisfaction of producing vegetables yourself, and the increased endorphins and physical activity will help your well-being.
- Expect more changes. Make healthy eating a habit, but accept that your tastes may change as your treatment, health and activity levels progress, so don't feel bound to one particular choice of diet.

Enjoy your food

Good food does more than provide nutrition. A tasty meal, particularly when shared with others, is enjoyable, making it good for the body and for the soul. Sometimes new routines can enhance that enjoyment.

- Relish your food. Take time to eat, savour and digest your meal.
- Show love and respect for food, life and self.
- Be aware of your environment when you eat. Try to make your surroundings pleasant, comfortable and relaxing.
- When you do allow yourself a treat, feel good about it; for example, focus on the beneficial aspects of the food, such as the antioxidants in coffee, red wine or chocolate, and know that the occasional treat can boost your endorphin levels, helping you to feel good.

The connection between food and mood

The food we eat alters the chemical balance of our bodies and affects our physical, emotional and spiritual health. Large and rapid ups and downs in the levels of blood glucose (sugar) are linked to changes in mood and energy. After a sugary snack, blood glucose can spike and then quite quickly drop again to a relatively low level. This can lead to irritability, light-headedness, lower concentration and tiredness, as in the "post-lunch dip". To help stabilize blood sugar levels, try some of the following:

- Eat regular meals. If you feel hungry, have a snack mid morning and/or afternoon.
- Combine protein, fat and fibre at each meal and snack. Eating low-GL meals (see page 13) helps to regulate the release of glucose and moderates mood. A protein-rich breakfast will help to reduce cravings later in the day.
- Drink plenty of fluids between meals. Brain function requires a large percentage of the body's intake of fluids, so have a glass of water near you to avoid dehydration. Avoid sugary drinks, sodas, fruit juices and too much tea or coffee.

• Include plenty of omega-3-rich foods to maintain a healthy brain, which is largely comprised of these fats. Omega-3 can also help to control insulin function.

Digestion and stress

Have you ever eaten a meal but barely tasted it? Or maybe had a snack without even registering it? Hasty, distracted eating when you are busy or stressed makes it difficult for your body to digest even the healthiest food.

How to improve your digestion

• Reduce stress when eating. A calming routine at mealtimes helps you to switch from your daily worries to the pleasure of eating. Take a little time (5–10 minutes) to sit down and stimulate your appetite to begin the digestive process. Try relaxation or imagery, or simply take two deep breaths before you eat. You may want to light a candle or put a vase of flowers on the table.

• Savour your food. Notice its colour and freshness, smell your food and enjoy its aroma, use as many of your senses as you can, even before you begin to eat. Taking time to anticipate meals prepares the digestive system.

• Eat slowly and mindfully. Chew every mouthful thoroughly, focusing on the nutrients, energy and pleasure your meal is giving you. This will stimulate your body to produce more enzymes and make digestion more efficient. If you are in the habit of eating quickly, try putting your knife and fork down between mouthfuls.

• Take a break. Let your digestive system rest between meals. Constant snacking is only necessary and useful if you have very poor blood sugar balance.

• Don't drink too much while eating, as this may dilute your digestive juices.

• Avoid eating late at night. This can raise insulin levels, increasing belly fat, and puts additional pressure on the digestive system as you try to sleep.

• Cook your food, if you are having digestion problems. Cooking food can help to break down some of the fibrous and tough material in the outer plant or animal membranes. Raw food, although nutritious and flavoursome, may be difficult to manage on occasions if your digestive system is affected by illness, treatments or drugs. Raw juices, however, do not contain fibre and are an easier way to get essential, concentrated nutrients than eating raw vegetables.

• Spice it up. Use spices or herbs with most meals (see page 20). Eating sour and/or bitter foods can help with any symptoms of indigestion you may have.

Natural condiments from the store-cupboard

There are lots of natural ingredients that you can add to dishes to create food bursting with flavours, and many of them possess powerful health-enhancing properties.

DEPTH AND RICHNESS	QUALITIES, BENEFITS	USE
Barley miso	Fermented soya and barley. Rich in phytoestrogens	Can be used for pungent salad dressings or for savoury dishes such as lentils or beans
Cacao powder, nibs, or cocoa	A naturally rich source of antioxidants and magnesium	Add 1 tbsp to chilli or lasagne. Adds depth to smoothies and sweet dishes
Sweet/white miso	Fermented soya and rice. Light in colour, texture and flavour. Rich in phytoestrogens	Suitable for salads and stir-fries. Delicious in marinades and soups
Tahini	A sesame paste rich in calcium, zinc and essential omega-6 fatty acids	Adds a nutty texture and flavour to dips, stir-fries, salads and dressings or as a spread on crackers

SAVOURY AND SALTY	QUALITIES, BENEFITS	USE
Anchovies	Can be used from a jar or tin. Add saltiness and bring out the flavour of other ingredients	Use as a whole garnish for salads or grain dishes. Can be crushed down into stir-fries and soups
Capers	Easy to source, available in jars. Rich in health-promoting flavonoids such as rutin and quercetin	Add a pungent and sour taste to dishes containing fish and grains
Nori/seaweed flakes	Rich in minerals and easy to use. Adds a slight saltiness to dishes. Good source of iodine	Can enhance the flavours of other ingredients. Great in soups, stews and added to salads
Nutritional yeast flakes	Inert yeast flakes in a carton. Rich in B vitamins. Give a yeasty/cheese flavour	Flavour balances well with nutmeg. Add to sauces and dressings. Great for flavouring vegan dishes
Pesto	Rich in flavour. Antioxidant benefits from its herb base	Add to stir-fries, pasta, potatoes, salad dressings and eggs
Tamari/shoyu	Good quality, naturally fermented soy sauces. Tamari is gluten-free	To add saltiness and depth. Use sparingly, as it is high in salt
Umeboshi vinegar/ume seasoning	An alkalizing fermented plum vinegar. Useful as a digestive aid	Add to stews, salads, stir-fries. Can be used in marinades
Wine/apple cider vinegar	Helps digestion and to stabilize blood glucose levels by reducing the glycaemic index/load	Choose a good-quality, naturally fermented vinegar. Add to salads, stews, stir-fries
Yeast extract	Rich in B vitamins (use in small amounts)	Adds pungency and saltiness to soups, casseroles and stir-fries

Although sugar should be as scant as possible in the diet, these healthier sweeteners have a lower glycaemic index than sugar, but it is still important to use them sparingly.

SWEETNESS	QUALITIES	USE
Apple juice concentrate (AJC)	Adds depth and balance to sweet and savoury dishes. High in fructose, so use sparingly	Useful for balancing the flavour of seaweed. Excellent in salads. Adds sweetness to a cake mixture
Lucuma	A nutrient-dense fruit from Peru, tasting like butterscotch	Use in ice creams and smoothies
Maca	A nutritious Peruvian root vegetable with a naturally sweet, caramel flavour. Used to modulate the effects of stress and to support hormonal health	Delicious added to drinks, cakes and desserts. Commonly found in powdered form
Molasses	A bitter edge to an overall sweetness. Can be quite dominant in taste. A high mineral content, including iron, calcium and magnesium	Use for sweet and savoury dishes. A little goes a long way
Stevia	A naturally sweet plant with a low glycaemic index	A little goes a long way. Supplied as granules
Xylitol	A natural sugar primarily derived from birch trees with minimal impact on blood sugar levels	Can be used like caster sugar, in cakes and puddings

Frequently Asked Questions

Why is organic food so important?

For some people, organic food is preferred for its better taste, or because of their concern for the environment; for others, it's their disquiet about the "cocktail" effect of multiple residues on human health. Safety standards exist for pesticide use in agriculture; however, where one additive may be safe in small amounts, this doesn't necessarily mean that in combination with others it is also safe. Organic foods are produced without the use of synthetic pesticides and chemical fertilizers. They do not contain genetically modified organisms and are not processed using irradiation, industrial solvents or chemical food additives.

A number of studies have indicated that there is a benefit to eating organic rather than industrially grown food in terms of safety (pesticide or chemical contamination and use of antibiotics), nutritional value, taste and environmental impact. It is, however, vital that you eat a variety of foods, rather than restricting your diet because you choose not to eat foods unless they are organically grown.

Wash all fruit and vegetables thoroughly with water. If using conventionally grown fruit and vegetables, adding a little vinegar or lemon juice to the washing water may help to remove surface chemicals, as will peeling.

If I don't eat dairy, what is the healthiest way to eat for strong bones?

Research is quite clear on this: those who eat plenty of fruit and vegetables daily have healthy bones. This is due to the alkalizing effect of fruit and vegetables, as well as due to the vitamin K, phytoestrogens and other bioactive nutrients found in abundance in these foods. Add to your diet small fish with bones, such as tinned sardines, as well as eating pulses, nuts and seeds (particularly sesame seeds and tahini), leafy green vegetables (such as cabbage, kale, spinach, parsley and watercress) and whole grains, all of which are rich in calcium. You get from these foods all the goodness that you need for your bones. Other dairy alternatives include:

- Oat, soya, rice and nut milks. Oat is particularly recommended, as it is easy to digest and usually free from added sugars.
- Healthy oils, such as olive oil or coconut oil, to spread or drizzle over bread.
- Alternatives to cheese include dips, pâtés and nut/seed butters.
- Soya yogurts are available; choose the unsweetened variety.
- Oat and nut creams are available.

Why should I reduce my coffee intake when it makes me feel so alert?

Caffeine is found in certain drinks such as tea (the black, green and white varieties) and especially coffee. It is also found in some foods such as chocolate. Caffeine can increase the body's production of stress hormones, including adrenaline, hence the feel-good factor. Increased adrenaline puts additional stress on the body's reserves of nutrients, however, and this process can also raise blood glucose levels. For this reason coffee is not recommended in large quantities or to be taken regularly. It is particularly important to minimize caffeine intake during times of stress. If you choose to drink coffee, do so in moderation and enjoy it.

Can I drink alcohol?

Some alcoholic drinks, such as red wine, contain compounds with beneficial antioxidant properties (for example, resveratrol). These properties are enhanced if organic products are used; however, alcohol itself offers very little benefit to the body, apart from its relaxation effects, and can place stress on the liver as well as undermining general health. Research evidence clearly shows that alcohol can increase the risk of certain cancers, as well as heart disease and high blood pressure.

If you choose to drink alcohol, ideally keep it for special occasions and celebrations, and enjoy it in moderation. Those having alcohol more regularly should not exceed one to two drinks a week. Antioxidant compounds similar to those in red wine can be obtained by eating a diet rich in fresh vegetables and fruit.

Would it be a good idea to become vegetarian or vegan?

Every individual has a different requirement for nutrients, and while some people thrive eating animal products, others don't, or choose to avoid them. We encourage people to eat a plant-based diet and avoid processed meat, but we do not recommend avoiding animal products completely, as they can contribute valuable, easily utilized protein and iron as well as other nutrients to the diet, including omega-3 fats (if the animals are grass fed and organic/free range), selenium, vitamins A and B12, and other B vitamins. If meat is particularly hard to digest, or undesirable, using small amounts of dairy – milk, yogurt and butter – and moderate amounts of eggs and fish would be advisable. If you choose to avoid animal products:

- Avoid restricting your food choices to just one or two foods to replace the protein and other nutrients present in animal products. A wide variety and combination of foods is essential, particularly if you are avoiding animal products. Seeds, nuts and pulses are all good sources of protein.
- Eat a variety of nutrient-rich plant foods to provide sufficient amino acids (the protein building blocks), vitamins, minerals and essential fatty acids. Plant sources with good profiles include: quinoa, buckwheat, amaranth, hemp seed and soya.
- Eat seaweeds, which contain vitamins, minerals, amino acids and iodine.
- Certain plant foods – pulses (peas and beans), whole grains and seeds – contain oxalate and phytate, which inhibit calcium absorption. Sprouting significantly reduces the phytate content, so using a combination of sprouted seeds and grains is beneficial. Phytates can also restrict iron absorption from plant foods (iron-rich foods include pulses, seeds and nuts). The inhibiting effect can be lessened by including vitamin C-rich foods in your diet.

Is it safe to eat soya?

Soya beans are a source of fibre, vitamins and minerals as well as phytoestrogens. Phytoestrogens, when obtained from a variety of plant foods and as part of a balanced diet, may have positive benefits for the body such as regulating certain hormones. Other sources of phytoestrogens include certain pulses, seeds, grains and vegetables. Phytoestrogens in food (rather than from supplements), don't seem to be a risk factor for cancer, so they do not need to be avoided. For vegetarians, soya products can provide a valuable source of complete protein. We do not, however, recommend the use of soya foods in large amounts (more than four servings weekly), because of the anti-nutrient factors (see page 21). Also, raw or sprouted soya beans may interfere with thyroid gland activity and should not be eaten by those with already compromised thyroid health. Cooked soya beans do not have the same effect.

Should I take supplements?

It is always better, if you can, to eat whole foods rather than taking supplements. The multiple bioactive components in food work together (synergistically), so that the combined effect is greater than the effect of the individual components.

However, alongside a healthy diet, and particularly if you are not able to eat sufficient quantities of food, you may wish to add a little extra nutritional support. If this is your choice:

• Always keep to recommended dosage instructions and take products designed for general nutritional support unless under professional guidance.

• Always inform your medical team of the supplements you are taking.

• Because there is still limited research on the use of supplements during treatments, we recommend you stop taking them during chemotherapy and radiotherapy, unless advised otherwise by your medical team.

7-Day Menu Plans

The following daily menus can be used as a basis when you plan your meals for the week. Mix and match as you like. You may also choose to minimize cooking by eating leftovers for lunch the next day or by cooking a larger quantity to eat another day.

Non-vegetarian

BREAKFAST	LUNCH	DINNER	SNACK
Mixed Seeded Granola, with yogurt (p.56)	Pan-Fried Squid with Red Cabbage & Walnuts (p.83)	Persian Quinoa Omega Bowl (p.117)	Ginger, Almond & Chocolate Cookies (p.141)
Spanish Baked Eggs (p.63)	Warm Lentil & Bean Salad (p.91)	Chicken & Cashew Nut Stir-Fry (p.94)	Coconut Rice Pudding (p.157)
Oat, Almond & Pear Porridge (p.144)	Garlic & Bean Soup with Pesto (p.71)	Baked Sea Bass with Olives & Tomatoes (p.103)	Baked Lemon Cheesecake (p.123)
Sardines with Roasted Tomatoes (p.65)	Wilted Kale Salad with Toasted Seeds (p.87)	Venison with Zesty Gremolata (p.101)	Wheatgrass Energizer (p.151)
Flaxseed, Apricot & Cinnamon Muffins (p.59)	Sicilian Prawns (p.82)	Spaghetti with Lemon & Broccoli (p.114)	Super-Berry Yogurt Sorbet (p.126)
Blueberry Avocado Build-Up Shake (p.142)	Noodle, Shallot & Shiitake Salad (p.148)	Turkey & Pistachio Korma (p.98)	Matcha Mango Shake (p.51)
Star Anise Poached Plums with Ginger Nut Cream (p.55)	Super-Greens Salad with Chicken (p.77)	Mixed Seafood Pie (p.109)	Italian Crackers & Bean Dip (p.158)

Vegetarian

BREAKFAST	LUNCH	DINNER	SNACK
Mixed Seeded Granola (p.56) with soya or coconut yogurt	Hoisin Tempeh Skewers (p.84)	Warm Aubergine, Roots & Chickpea Salad (p.113)	Coconut Rice Pudding (p.157)
Spiced Flatbreads (p.135), with hummus or nut butter	Creamy Cauliflower Soup (p.72)	Hemp Seed & Nut Burgers (p.116), Celeriac, Apple & Fennel Remoulade (p.88)	Stamina-Boosting Beetroot Juice (p.151)
Green Hemp Shake (p.51), Date & Lucuma Cocoa Bar (p.60)	Pepper Bisque with Chilli Cream (p.74)	Roasted Tempeh with Piperade Sauce (p.110)	Matcha Tea & Banana Cake (p.130)
Date & Lucuma Cocoa Bar (p.60)	Garlic & Bean Soup with Pesto (p.71)	Persian Quinoa Omega Bowl (p.117)	Super-Berry Yogurt Sorbet (p.126)
Star Anise Poached Plums with Ginger Nut Cream (p.55)	Mixed Sea Vegetable & Cucumber Salad (p.90)	Spaghetti with Lemon & Broccoli (p.114)	Coconut Cocoa Booster (p.154)
Oat, Almond & Pear Porridge (p.144)	Super-Greens Salad with Nut Dressing (p.76)	Red Cabbage & Walnuts (p.83), Italian Crackers & Bean Dip (p.158)	Chocolate Beetroot Traybake (p.133)
Flaxseed, Apricot & Cinnamon Muffins (p.59)	Wilted Kale Salad with Toasted Seeds (p.87)	Warm Lentil & Bean Salad (p.91), Spiced Flatbreads (p.135)	Baked Lemon Cheesecake (p.123)

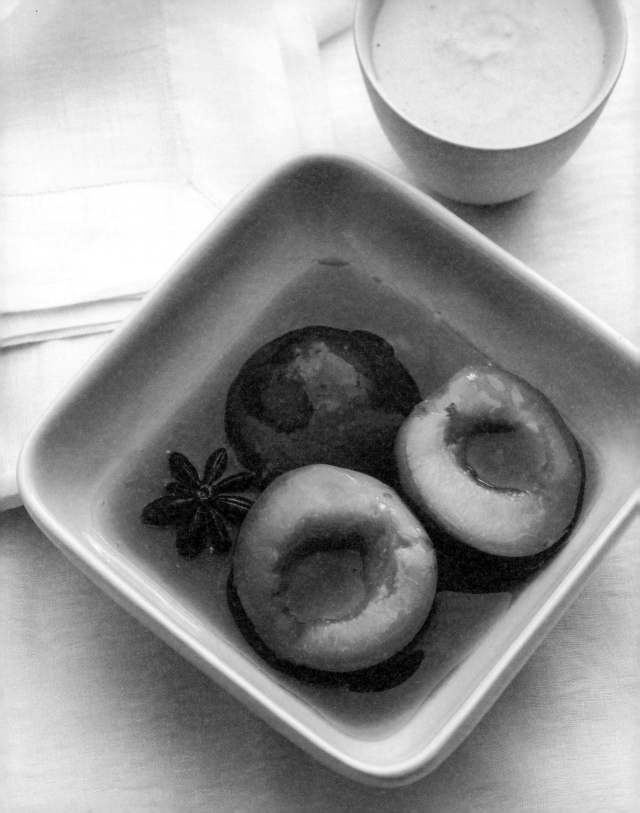

Shakes, Juices, Smoothies & Breakfasts

A shake, juice or smoothie contains beneficial ingredients in a form that is easy to take, making it useful for breakfast or as a snack, particularly if you find your appetite is low or you're just too tired to cook a meal. Other tempting breakfast options in this chapter include Flaxseed, Apricot & Cinnamon Muffins, omega-rich Mixed Seeded Granola, warming Star Anise Poached Plums with Ginger Nut Cream, and speedy Spanish Baked Eggs. Whether it's a quick pick-me-up you need or something to keep you going during treatment, the recipes in this chapter are packed with nutrients to support your body and are designed to reinvigorate your appetite, bolster your energy levels and kick-start your metabolism.

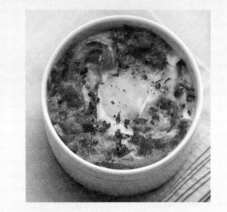

Opposite: Star Anise Poached Plums with Ginger Nut Cream (page 54)
Above: Spanish Baked Eggs (page 62)

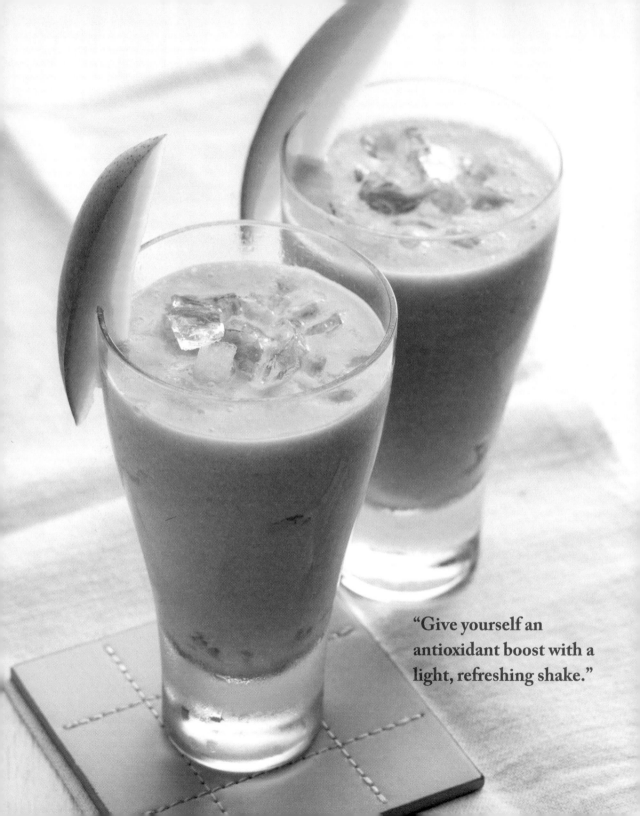

"Give yourself an antioxidant boost with a light, refreshing shake."

◂ Matcha Mango Shake

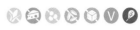

1 Put the almonds in a blender or food processor with 500ml/17fl oz/2 cups water and process until smooth. Strain through a fine sieve, if you prefer.

2 Add the mango and the matcha, and process again until thick and creamy. Drink immediately, served with ice and mango, if you like, or store in the fridge for up to 2 days.

SERVES 2, 250ml/9fl oz/1 cup each
PREPARATION TIME 5 minutes

60g/2¼oz/heaped ⅓ cup blanched almonds
1 ripe mango, peeled, pitted and diced
1 tsp matcha green tea
ice, to serve
mango slices, to serve (optional)

NUTRITIONAL INFORMATION PER SERVING
Protein 9.4g, **Carbohydrates** 11.8g of which sugars 11.1g, **Fat** 16.9g of which saturates 1.4g, **Kcals** 234

HEALTH BENEFITS
Matcha is an antioxidant-rich powdered Japanese green tea. The whole leaves are used, making matcha more potent than brewed green tea and higher in antioxidants.

Green Hemp Shake

1 Put all the ingredients into a blender or food processor and process until smooth. Drink immediately or store in the fridge for up to 1 day.

SERVES 2, 250ml/9fl oz/1 cup each
PREPARATION TIME 5 minutes

30g/1oz/¼ cup hemp protein powder or shelled hemp seeds
1 ripe mango, peeled, pitted and diced
a pinch of cinnamon
400ml/14fl oz/generous 1½ cups coconut water or water
2 large handfuls of spinach leaves, romaine lettuce or kale
a pinch of stevia, if needed, to taste

NUTRITIONAL INFORMATION PER SERVING
Protein 10g, **Carbohydrates** 19.9g of which sugars 10.3g, **Fats** 2.6g of which saturates 0.1g, **Kcals** 142

HEALTH BENEFITS
Hemp protein powder is an easy and healthy way to increase your intake of quality protein and omega-3 and -6 essential fats. It also helps to stabilize blood sugar levels.

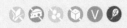

Green Elixir

SERVES 1, 250ml/9fl oz/1 cup
PREPARATION TIME 5 minutes

2 celery sticks
½ cucumber
2 large handfuls of kale
2cm/¾in piece of fresh root ginger
1 lemon
2 apples
ice cubes, to serve (optional)
1 tbsp seeds or nuts, to serve

1 Put all the ingredients through an electric juicer and drink immediately or store in the fridge for up to 1 day. Serve with ice, if you like, and with 1 tablespoon seeds or nuts.

NUTRITIONAL INFORMATION PER SERVING
Protein 3.6g, **Carbohydrates** 19.9g of which sugars 18.6g,
Fat 1.2g of which saturates 0.1g, **Kcals** 100

HEALTH BENEFITS
This light and cleansing juice contains ginger to ease nausea and digestive upsets. (If you have thyroid problems, limit your intake of brassicas such as raw kale, as they can have a goitrogenic effect, lowering the function of the thyroid and reducing metabolism.)

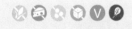

Digestive Healer

SERVES 1, 250ml/9fl oz/1 cup
PREPARATION TIME 5 minutes

½ pineapple, peeled (core included)
1cm/½in piece of fresh root ginger
1 handful of parsley
100g/3½oz baby spinach leaves
½ cucumber
1 tbsp aloe vera juice (optional)
1 tbsp seeds or nuts, to serve

1 Put the pineapple, ginger, parsley and vegetables through an electric juicer. Add the aloe vera juice, if using, and stir to combine. Drink immediately or store in the fridge for up to 1 day. Serve with 1 tablespoon seeds or nuts.

NUTRITIONAL INFORMATION PER SERVING
Protein 8.9g, **Carbohydrates** 33.8g of which sugars 32.8g,
Fat 8.6g of which saturates 1.2g, **Kcals** 250

HEALTH BENEFITS
Aloe vera is a known digestive aid and it is combined here with digestion-supporting ginger. Cucumber is hydrating and a source of antioxidants.

Brazil Nut Cream

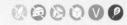

1 Put the nuts in a blender or food processor with 400ml/
  14fl oz/generous 1½ cups water and process until smooth.
  Add the remaining ingredients and process again. Drink
  immediately or store in the fridge for up to 1 day.

SERVES 2, 250ml/9fl oz/1 cup each
PREPARATION TIME 5 minutes

60g/2¼oz/heaped ⅓ cup Brazil nuts
200g/7oz fresh or frozen strawberries
½ tsp vanilla extract
2 tsp lecithin granules (optional)

NUTRITIONAL INFORMATION PER SERVING
Protein 5.1g, **Carbohydrates** 6.4g of which sugars 6.4g,
Fat 20.6g of which saturates 5.2g, **Kcals** 247

HEALTH BENEFITS
This smoothie contains protein and healthy fats. Brazil nuts are one of the most
concentrated sources of selenium, which is important for protecting cells from damage.

Redbush Apricot Cream

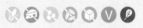

1 Put the tea bag in a jug and pour over 250ml/9fl oz/1 cup
  boiling water. Leave to soak for 10 minutes, then remove
  the tea bag and discard. Leave to cool slightly.
2 Put the remaining ingredients into a blender or food
  processor and pour over the tea. Process until smooth.
  Drink immediately or store in the fridge for up to 1 day.
  Serve cold or warm.

SERVES 1, 250ml/9fl oz/1 cup
PREPARATION TIME 5 minutes,
  plus 10 minutes soaking

1 redbush (rooibos) tea bag
2 fresh apricots, cut in half and stoned, or
  4 tinned apricot halves, in natural juice
40g/1½oz/¼ cup cashew nuts
30g/1oz/scant ¼ cup ready-to-eat dried
  apricots

NUTRITIONAL INFORMATION PER SERVING
Protein 9.3g, **Carbohydrates** 22.3g of which sugars 17.7g,
Fat 19.5g of which saturates 3.8g, **Kcals** 301

HEALTH BENEFITS
Redbush tea, from the South African rooibos plant, is caffeine-free and low in tannins. It is
also extremely rich in antioxidants including the flavonoids quercetin and luteolin.

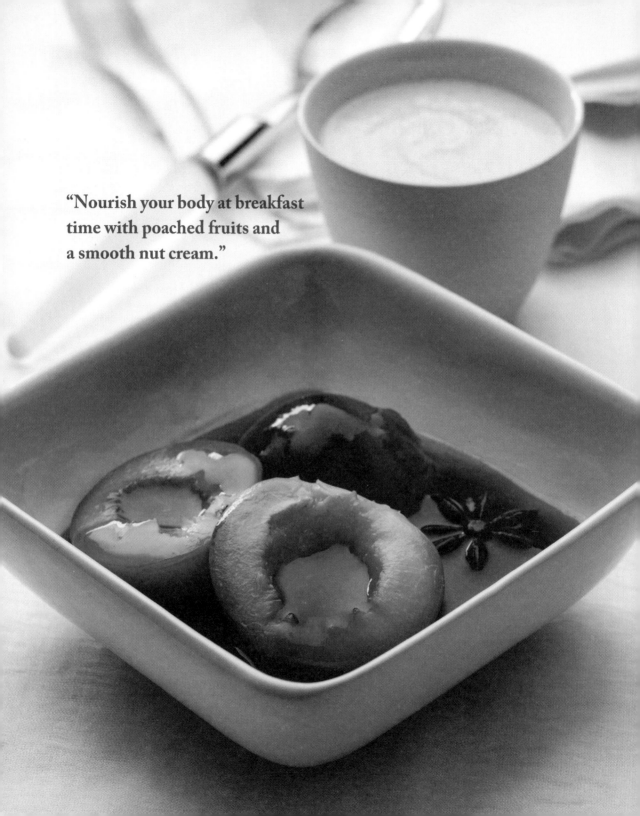

"Nourish your body at breakfast time with poached fruits and a smooth nut cream."

Star Anise Poached Plums with Ginger Nut Cream

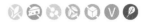

Plums are poached in lightly spiced pomegranate juice then topped with a ginger nut cream. The plums can be served hot or left to soak in the scented juice and served cold. This is a useful recipe for making in a batch to serve for breakfasts or snacks over 2 to 3 days.

1 Put the plums, pomegranate juice, star anise and cinnamon stick in a saucepan. Bring to the boil, then lower the heat and simmer for 5 minutes or until the fruit is just soft. Mix the cornflour with 1 tablespoon water and add to the pan, stirring until thickened. Leave to cool to develop the flavours.

2 To make the ginger nut cream, put all the ingredients into a blender or food processor and process until smooth. Add a little water, if necessary.

3 Discard the cinnamon stick and the star anise, and serve the plums either warm or cold with the ginger nut cream. (Store in the fridge for up to 3 days.)

SERVES 4
PREPARATION TIME 10 minutes
COOKING TIME 6 minutes, plus
   cooling

6 large or 8 medium red plums, cut in half
   and pitted
250ml/9fl oz/1 cup pure pomegranate
   juice
2 star anise
1 cinnamon stick
2 tsp cornflour or arrowroot

Ginger nut cream
125g/4½oz/heaped ¾ cup cashew nuts
2 tbsp olive oil or coconut oil
125ml/4fl oz/½ cup fresh orange juice
2cm/¾in piece fresh root ginger, peeled
   and grated

NUTRITIONAL INFORMATION PER SERVING
Protein 6.3g, **Carbohydrates** 22.6g of which sugars 16.6g, **Fat** 22.7g of which saturates 9.5g, **Kcals** 320

HEALTH BENEFITS
Fresh and dried plums (prunes) contain disease-protective phytonutrients, and the high fibre of prunes has a mild laxative effect aiding bowel function and regularity. Plums are rich in phenols and vitamin C, which can assist with the absorption of iron. Vitamin C is needed in the body to make healthy tissue and support the immune system. The ginger nut cream provides protein and healthy fats, with the addition of fresh ginger, which helps to support the digestion and ease the symptoms of nausea.

Mixed Seeded Granola

SERVES 8
PREPARATION TIME 10 minutes
COOKING TIME 50 minutes

115g/4oz/scant 1¼ cups rolled oats
60g/2¼oz/heaped ⅓ cup almonds,
 chopped
60g/2¼oz/ heaped ⅓ cup Brazil nuts,
 chopped
2 tbsp chia seeds (optional)
4 tbsp shelled hemp seeds
60g/2¼oz/½ cup sunflower seeds
60g/2¼oz/½ cup pumpkin seeds
60g/2¼oz/heaped ⅓ cup sesame seeds
1 tbsp xylitol or ½ tsp stevia (optional)
2 tbsp olive oil or melted coconut oil
1 pear, chopped
1 tsp cinnamon
½ tsp ground ginger
4 tbsp apple juice
60g/2¼oz/½ cup dried unsweetened
 berries of your choice
30g/1oz/⅓ cup goji berries

The omega-3 fats in this protein- and nutrient-dense crunchy cereal have been preserved through baking the granola in a low oven. Serve the granola for breakfast with yogurt or milk, or a milk alternative, or use as a snack or topping for fruit dishes.

1 Preheat the oven to 160°C/315°F/Gas 2½ and line a baking sheet with baking parchment. Put the oats, nuts and seeds in a bowl and mix thoroughly. Put the remaining ingredients, except the berries, into a blender or food processor and process until smooth.

2 Pour the wet mixture over the oats, and combine thoroughly with your hands to ensure the oats and nuts are evenly coated.

3 Spread the mixture on to the prepared baking sheet. Bake for 45–50 minutes until golden and crisp. Leave the granola to cool, then stir in the dried berries. Serve. (Store in an airtight container for 1–2 weeks.)

NUTRITIONAL INFORMATION PER SERVING
Protein 11.3g, **Carbohydrates** 24.4g of which sugars 11g, **Fat** 27.2g of which saturates 5.6g, **Kcals** 387

HEALTH BENEFITS
Shelled hemp seeds are easily digestible and a complete protein source. They also contain high amounts of fatty acids and fibre, trace minerals and vitamin E. The Brazil nuts are selenium rich and the sunflower and pumpkin seeds are plentiful in omega-6 essential fats.

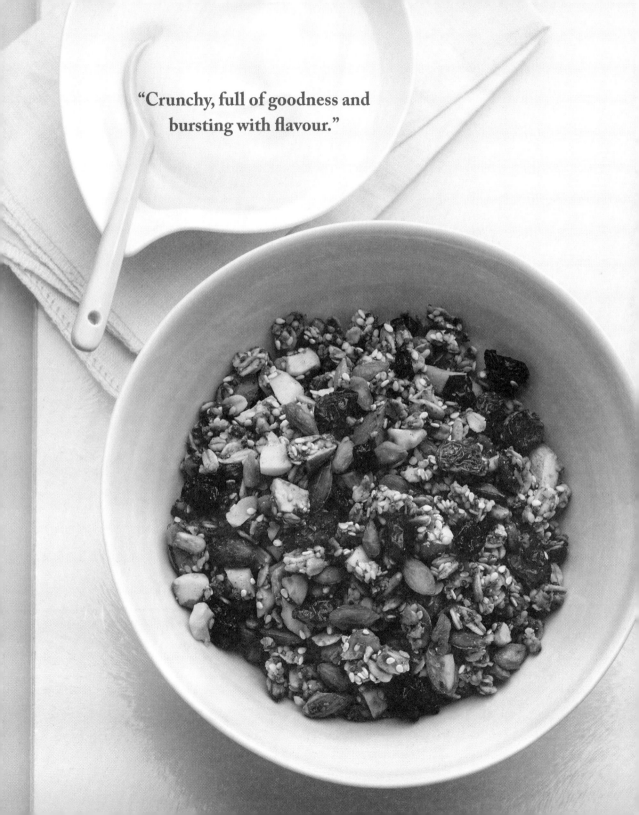

"Crunchy, full of goodness and bursting with flavour."

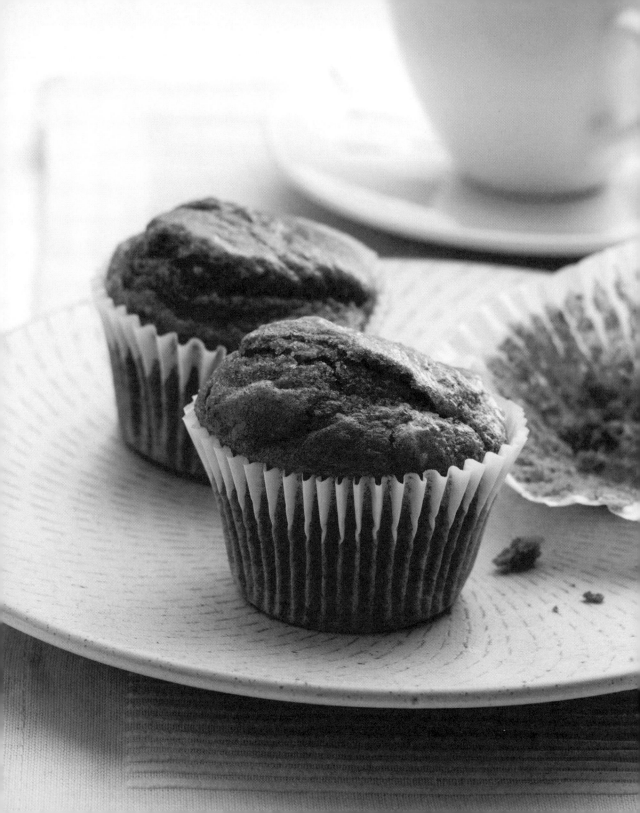

Flaxseed, Apricot & Cinnamon Muffins

These muffins, sweetened with fruit, are rich in soluble fibre thanks to the addition of ground flaxseed. Choose them for a breakfast treat or a healthy snack to keep your energy levels high throughout the day.

MAKES 10
PREPARATION TIME 15 minutes
COOKING TIME 25 minutes, plus cooling

1 Preheat the oven to 180°C/350°F/Gas 4. Line 10 muffin cups with paper cases or grease the cups. In a large bowl, sift together the flour, baking powder, bicarbonate of soda, salt and cinnamon. Tip in any bran left in the sieve, then mix in the xylitol and flaxseed.

2 In a jug or blender, mix together the oil, juice, yogurt and eggs. Add to the flour mixture and beat with a wooden spoon to form a smooth, thick batter.

3 Stir in the apricots and ginger. Fill each muffin cup about three-quarters full. Bake for 20–25 minutes until a skewer inserted into the centre comes out clean. Leave the muffins to cool for a few minutes before removing to a wire rack to cool completely before serving. (Store in the fridge for up to 3 days or freeze for up to 1 month.)

4 tbsp olive oil, plus extra for greasing, if needed
225g/8oz/1½ cups wholemeal plain flour or gluten-free flour mix
2 tsp baking powder
1 tsp bicarbonate of soda
a pinch of sea salt
1½ tsp cinnamon
2 tbsp xylitol
3 tbsp ground flaxseed
125ml/4fl oz/½ cup apple juice
225g/8oz/scant 1 cup natural yogurt or soya yogurt
3 eggs
60g/2¼oz/⅓ cup ready-to-eat dried apricots, chopped
2cm/¾in piece fresh root ginger, peeled and grated

NUTRITIONAL INFORMATION PER MUFFIN
Protein 5.7g, **Carbohydrates** 26.8g of which sugars 8.9g, **Fat** 5g of which saturates 1.9g, **Kcals** 173

HEALTH BENEFITS
Dried apricots contain soluble fibre to help bowel health. Their high beta-carotene content is converted by the body into vitamin A, which is a powerful antioxidant, quenching free-radical damage to cells and tissues and supporting immune health. Fresh root ginger is a warming spice that is frequently used to support the digestion and calm the feelings of nausea. Ground cinnamon helps to balance blood sugar levels.

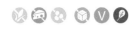

Date & Lucuma Cocoa Bars

MAKES 16

PREPARATION TIME 15 minutes,
plus 10 minutes soaking and at least
1 hour chilling

140g/5oz/¾ cup pitted dried dates

115g/4oz/heaped 1 cup pecan nuts

115g/4oz/scant 1 cup walnut pieces

30g/1oz/¼ cup cocoa powder or
cacao powder

4 tbsp shelled hemp seeds

60g/2¼oz/scant ½ cup lucuma powder

2 tbsp chia seeds or ground flaxseed

zest and juice of 1 lemon

75g/2½oz/scant ½ cup cashew or almond
nut butter

Lucuma powder is made from a nutrient-dense fruit from Peru, which is traditionally used in ice creams and desserts, and has a maple syrup flavour. Enjoy these healthy raw bars for breakfast or as a snack, straight from the fridge, or in a lunch box (although they will be a little softer when eaten at room temperature).

1 Soak the dates in hot water for 10 minutes, then drain and set aside. Line a 20cm/8in square shallow traybake tin with baking parchment. Put the nuts in a blender or food processor and process until very finely ground. Transfer to a bowl and add the cocoa powder, hemp seeds, lucuma powder and chia seeds.

2 Put the dates, lemon zest and juice into a blender or food processor with the nut butter and process to form a thick paste. Add to the bowl and use your hands to combine the mixture into a soft dough.

3 Press the mixture into the prepared tin. Put into the fridge and chill for 1–2 hours to firm up, or freeze for 1 hour. Cut into bars to serve. (Store, individually wrapped, in the fridge for up to 1 week or freeze for up to 1 month.)

NUTRITIONAL INFORMATION PER BAR
Protein 4.4g, **Carbohydrates** 11.6g of which sugars 6.7g, **Fat** 14.3g of which saturates 1.6g, **Kcals** 194

HEALTH BENEFITS
Dates are a great way to add a natural sweetness to dishes, and their soluble fibre slows down the release of sugars in the body to keep you energized for longer. Lucuma is a useful low-glycaemic natural sweetener. It also provides fibre, vitamins and minerals, including beta-carotene, niacin (B3) and iron.

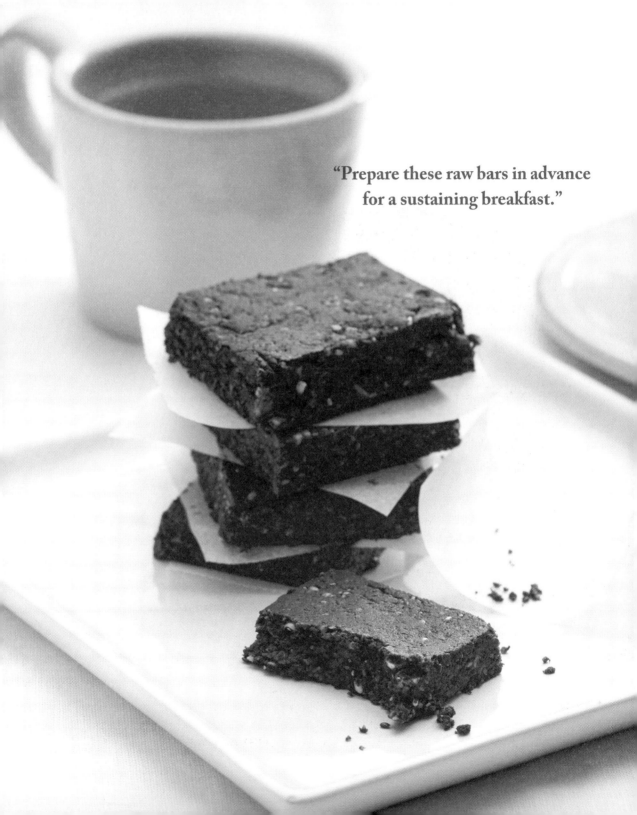

"Prepare these raw bars in advance for a sustaining breakfast."

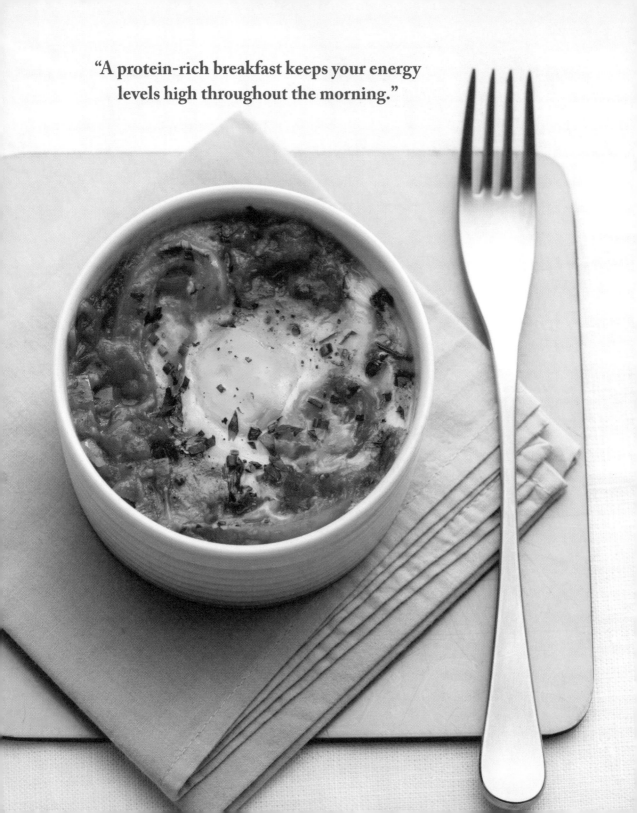

"A protein-rich breakfast keeps your energy levels high throughout the morning."

Spanish Baked Eggs

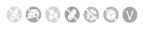

This rustic Spanish-inspired breakfast or brunch-style dish combines antioxidant-rich peppers and tomatoes with herbs. It can be mostly prepared in advance – just crack in the eggs when ready to cook. Although the recipe calls for 1 egg per person, you could add more eggs or a tin of chickpeas, drained and rinsed, to the vegetables.

1 Preheat the oven to 160°C/315°F/Gas 2½. Heat the olive oil in a frying pan over low heat – preferably using an ovenproof frying pan – and add the onion, peppers, garlic and spices. Cook gently for 10 minutes or until the peppers are soft.

2 Add the tomatoes and simmer for 1–2 minutes until the sauce has thickened. Stir in the lemon juice and scatter over the herbs.

3 If necessary, transfer the vegetables to a shallow baking dish or individual ramekins. Make four indents into the mixture, or one for each ramekin, and crack in the eggs. Season with pepper. Bake for 6–8 minutes until the whites are fully set but the yolks are still a little runny. Serve hot, sprinkled with herbs. (Store in the fridge for up to 1 day.)

SERVES 4
PREPARATION TIME 10 minutes
COOKING TIME 20 minutes

2 tbsp olive oil
1 red onion, finely chopped
1 red pepper, deseeded and cut into strips
1 yellow pepper, deseeded and cut into strips
2 garlic cloves, crushed
½ tsp harissa paste, or to taste
½ tsp smoked paprika
400g/14oz/scant 1⅔ cups tinned chopped tomatoes
2 tbsp lemon juice
1 tbsp chopped parsley leaves, plus extra to serve
1 tbsp chopped chives, plus extra to serve
4 eggs
freshly ground black pepper

NUTRITIONAL INFORMATION PER SERVING
Protein 8.7g, **Carbohydrates** 9.9g of which sugars 8.9g, **Fat** 10.5g of which saturates 2.3g, **Kcals** 169

HEALTH BENEFITS
Garlic contains potent anti-microbial and anti-cancer phytonutrients. Peppers, and particularly red peppers, are one of the best sources of vitamin C, which strengthens the immune cells. There is about 250mg vitamin C in a large red pepper. The folic acid in the egg yolks is important for the replication of DNA and also protects the DNA during radiotherapy.

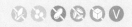

Turkish Breakfast

SERVES 2
PREPARATION TIME 5 minutes
COOKING TIME 15 minutes

3 vine-ripened tomatoes, cut in half
1 courgette, thickly sliced on the diagonal
2 tbsp olive oil
1 garlic clove, finely chopped
2 tsp chopped oregano
2 eggs
60g/2¼oz/½ cup pitted black olives
60g/2¼oz feta cheese, crumbled
sea salt and freshly ground black pepper

A filling summery dish of Mediterranean roasted tomatoes and courgette flavoured with oregano and garlic, and accented with olives. Feta cheese and egg provide protein to accompany the vegetables. It makes an ideal late-morning breakfast. Serve with 2 eggs per person, if you are avoiding dairy.

1 Preheat the oven to 180°C/350°F/Gas 4. Put the tomatoes, cut side up, into a baking dish and add the courgette. Drizzle over the oil and scatter over the garlic and oregano. Season with salt and pepper. Roast for 15 minutes or until soft.

2 Meanwhile, pour boiling water into a frying pan to a depth of 2.5cm/1in. Return to the boil then reduce to a simmer. Break the eggs into the water and poach for 6–8 minutes until the whites are firm but the yolk is a little runny. Toss the olives and cheese into the vegetables, and serve with the poached eggs. (Store in the fridge for up to 1 day.)

NUTRITIONAL INFORMATION PER SERVING
Protein 13.3g, **Carbohydrates** 4.6g of which sugars 4.5g, **Fat** 19.9g of which saturates 7g, **Kcals** 251

HEALTH BENEFITS
Eggs are an economical way to boost your protein intake. One egg contains about 6g of complete high-quality protein. Eggs are also a useful source of choline – the key component of many fat-containing structures in cell membranes, making it particularly important for brain function and health.

Sardines with Roasted Tomatoes

Oven-roasting the tomatoes intensifies their sweet flavour as well as contributing to the nutritional value of this ultra-healthy breakfast choice. Serve with sourdough or rye bread.

1 Preheat the oven to 190°C/375°F/Gas 5. Stir the garlic into the olive oil.
2 Put the tomatoes on a baking tray and pour over the garlic oil. Season with salt and pepper. Roast for 10 minutes or until the tomatoes are soft but still holding their shape.
3 Add the spinach leaves and lemon juice, and gently mix with the tomatoes, then roast for a further 5 minutes. Sprinkle over the pine nuts and serve with the sardines. (If you prefer, the sardines can be added to the dish with the spinach for the final 5 minutes of cooking.) (Store in the fridge for up to 1 day.)

SERVES 4
PREPARATION TIME 5 minutes
COOKING TIME 15 minutes

2 garlic cloves, crushed
2 tbsp olive oil or melted coconut oil
200g/7oz/1⅓ cups cherry tomatoes
200g/7oz baby leaf spinach
1 tsp lemon juice
60g/2¼oz/heaped ⅓ cup pine nuts or
   sunflower seeds
240g/8½oz tinned sardines in water or
   olive oil, drained
sea salt and freshly ground black pepper

NUTRITIONAL INFORMATION PER SERVING
Protein 20.1g, **Carbohydrates** 2.9g of which sugars 2.8g, **Fat** 22.6g of which saturates 4.7g, **Kcals** 295

HEALTH BENEFITS
Serving cooked tomatoes with omega-3-rich oily fish helps to facilitate the absorption of lycopene, an important phytonutrient found in tomatoes, which has been shown to be protective against certain forms of cancer. Vitamin- and mineral-rich spinach is a valuable energizing addition to the dish.

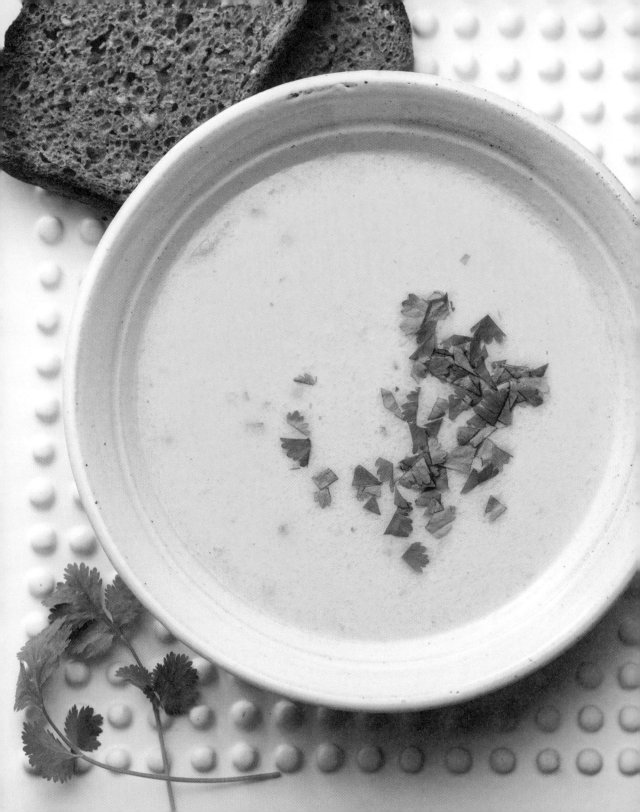

Soups & Light Dishes

When your energy levels and appetite are low, soups and light dishes that are quick and easy to assemble, yet nourishing, are the perfect solution. Simply prepared nutrient-packed broths, or light meat, fish or vegetarian dishes, will cram in plenty of foods capable of soothing and healing the body. The soups and light meals in this chapter are a step away from the ordinary, including a sensational dairy-free, creamy Broccoli & Cashew Nut Soup, and a quick-and-easy prawn dish from Sicily. All the recipes focus on using key foods and ingredients that have been shown to help recovery from cancer, promote immune health, reduce inflammation and aid healing, and many can be prepared in advance. If you choose not to eat animal products, several of the recipes can be adapted using vegetable protein.

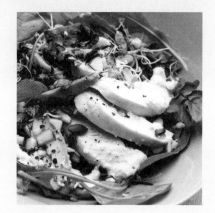

Opposite: Creamy Cauliflower Soup (page 72)
Above: Super-Greens Salad with Chicken (page 76)

Broccoli & Cashew Nut Soup

SERVES 4
PREPARATION TIME 20 minutes
COOKING TIME 6 minutes

1l/35fl oz/4 cups vegetable stock
2 garlic cloves, crushed
1cm/½in piece fresh root ginger, peeled
  and grated
60g/2¼oz/heaped ⅓ cup cashew nuts
1 tsp Thai fish sauce
1 tbsp apple cider vinegar
1 tbsp tamari, plus extra for drizzling
500g/1lb 2oz broccoli, cut into small
  pieces
1 tbsp olive oil or walnut oil
sea salt and freshly ground black pepper

A velvety soup that is particularly appealing when your appetite is low or if you're looking for a well-rounded meal in a bowl. It has a hint of Asian flavourings, including the salty, tangy flavour of Thai fish sauce, which complements the flavour of the cashew nuts. Serve with wholemeal or rye bread.

1 Put the stock, garlic, ginger, cashew nuts, fish sauce, vinegar and tamari into a large saucepan and bring to the boil. Add the broccoli and simmer for 2 minutes or until the broccoli is just tender.

2 Process the soup in a blender or food processor until smooth and thick. Add the oil and process again to combine. Season with salt and pepper. Serve drizzled with a little tamari to taste. (Store in the fridge for up to 3 days or freeze for 1 month.)

NUTRITIONAL INFORMATION PER SERVING
Protein 8.5g, **Carbohydrates** 5.2g of which sugars 2.8g, **Fat** 12.3g of which saturates 2g, **Kcals** 167

HEALTH BENEFITS
The combination of broccoli, garlic and ginger provides nutrients and phytochemicals that modulate immune function and reduce excess inflammation.

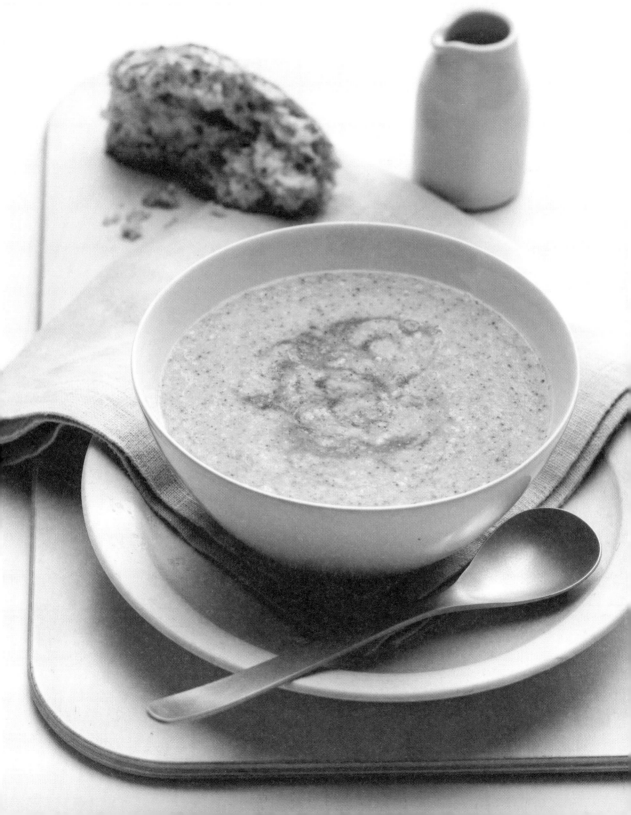

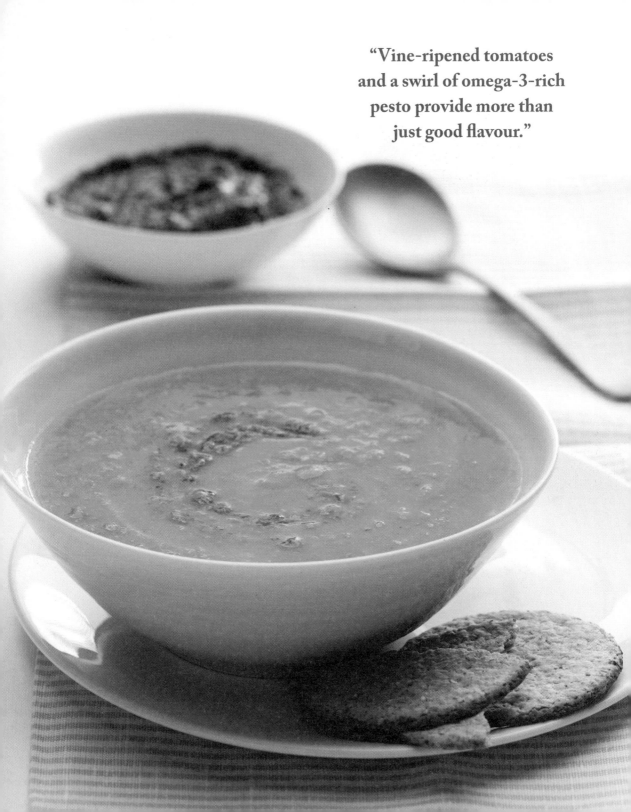

"Vine-ripened tomatoes and a swirl of omega-3-rich pesto provide more than just good flavour."

Garlic & Bean Soup with Pesto

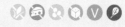

Roasting the garlic and tomatoes creates a naturally sweet and caramelized flavour to this Mediterranean-style soup. The tangy lemony pesto for the topping can be prepared in advance and stored in the fridge. You can also thin it down with a little vegetable stock to make a sauce for drizzling over vegetables and grains. Serve with oatcakes.

1 Preheat the oven to 200°C/400°F/Gas 6. Put the garlic cloves in a roasting tin, add the olive oil and toss to coat. Roast for 15 minutes. Add the tomatoes and roast for 10–15 minutes until the garlic is lightly golden and the tomatoes are soft.

2 Put the garlic, tomatoes, beans and stock into a blender or food processor and process until smooth. Pour into a saucepan and heat gently until warmed through. Add the lemon juice and season with salt and pepper.

3 To make the pesto, put the nuts and seeds in a food processor and process until finely ground. Add the herbs, garlic, yeast flakes, if using, lemon juice and a pinch of salt, and process. Drizzle in the oil with the machine running, to create a thick pesto. Serve the soup with a spoonful of pesto. (Store the soup in the fridge for up to 3 days. Store the pesto in the fridge for up to 1 week.)

SERVES 4

PREPARATION TIME 10 minutes

COOKING TIME 35 minutes

1 garlic bulb, cloves peeled

2 tbsp olive oil

450g/1lb vine-ripened tomatoes, cut into quarters

400g/14oz/2 cups tinned borlotti or kidney beans, drained and rinsed

700ml/24floz/generous 2¾ cups vegetable stock

1 tbsp lemon juice

sea salt and freshly ground black pepper

Pumpkin seed pesto

30g/1oz/¼ cup shelled pistachio nuts

30g/1oz/¼ cup pumpkin seeds

2 large handfuls of basil leaves

1 handful of mint leaves

1 garlic clove, crushed

2 tbsp nutritional yeast flakes (optional)

1 tbsp lemon juice

2–3 tbsp olive oil or walnut oil

NUTRITIONAL INFORMATION PER SERVING
Protein 5.9g, **Carbohydrates** 13.7g of which sugars 5.5g, **Fat** 3.9g of which saturates 0.5g, **Kcals** 116

HEALTH BENEFITS
Tomatoes have a plentiful supply of antioxidants and phytonutrients, which are protective against certain forms of cancer. One, alpha-tomatine, has been linked to prostate cancer prevention, and the carotenoid lycopene may help protect against breast cancer. The pesto is packed with essential omega-3 fats, zinc from the pumpkin seeds and mint to aid digestion.

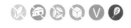

Creamy Cauliflower Soup

SERVES 4
PREPARATION TIME 10 minutes
COOKING TIME 20 minutes

1 tbsp olive oil or coconut oil
1 onion, finely chopped
3 garlic cloves, roughly chopped
1 red chilli, deseeded and diced (optional)
½ tsp turmeric
1 large head of cauliflower, cut into florets
400ml/14fl oz/generous 1½ cups tinned
    coconut milk
600ml/21fl oz/scant 2½ cups vegetable
    stock
2 tsp tamari
freshly ground black pepper
1 handful of coriander leaves, chopped,
    to serve

A soothing dairy-free soup with a coconut base and a little spicy kick from garlic and chilli. The soup can be prepared in advance and reheated. Serve with toasted wholegrain rye or pumpernickel bread.

1 Heat the oil in a large saucepan over medium heat and gently fry the onion, garlic, chilli, if using, and turmeric for 5 minutes. Add the cauliflower florets and stir to coat in the oil.

2 Pour in the coconut milk, stock and tamari. Bring to the boil, then lower the heat and simmer gently for 15 minutes or until the cauliflower is soft. Season to taste with pepper.

3 Process the soup in a blender or food processor until smooth. Serve sprinkled with chopped coriander leaves. (Store in the fridge for up to 3 days or freeze for 1 month.)

NUTRITIONAL INFORMATION PER SERVING
Protein 4.7g, **Carbohydrate** 10.7g of which sugars 9.3g, **Fat** 3.8g of which saturates 2.4g, **Kcals** 95

HEALTH BENEFITS
The compound curcumin, present in turmeric, has cancer-protective, anti-inflammatory properties, and the chilli contains capsaicin, also known for its anti-cancer properties. Cauliflower is a cruciferous vegetable that is rich in phytonutrients called glucosinolates, which can help to activate detoxification enzymes and reduce the toxic burden on the body. It is rich in antioxidants including vitamin C, manganese and phytonutrients as well as vitamin K known for its anti-inflammatory properties.

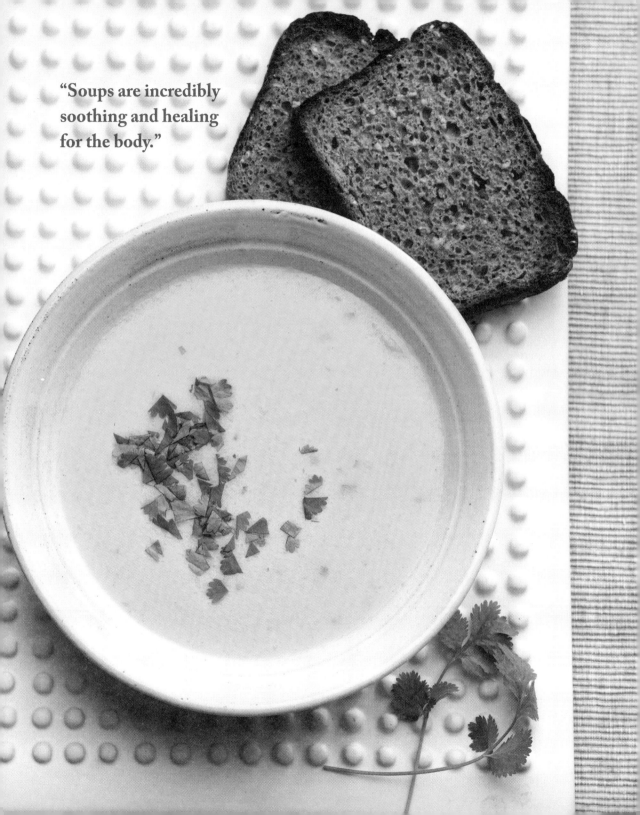

"Soups are incredibly soothing and healing for the body."

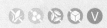

Pepper Bisque with Chilli Cream

SERVES 4

PREPARATION TIME 10 minutes

COOKING TIME 25 minutes, plus cooling and chilling

3 red peppers, cut in half and deseeded
1 tbsp olive oil or coconut oil
1 red onion, finely chopped
1 garlic clove, crushed
a pinch of crushed chillies (optional)
600ml/21fl oz/scant 2½ cups vegetable stock
400g/14oz/2 cups tinned cannellini beans, drained and rinsed

Chilli cream
100g/3½oz/heaped ⅓ cup Greek yogurt
1 red chilli, deseeded and finely chopped
2 tbsp roughly chopped basil leaves

Cannellini beans add protein to this chilled summer soup topped with a little chilli-infused yogurt, although the chilli can be omitted if you prefer. The soup is also excellent served hot. Serve with sourdough or oatcakes.

1 Preheat the grill. Put the peppers cut side down on a baking tray and grill until the skin has blackened all over. Transfer to a bowl, cover with cling film and leave to cool for 10 minutes. Peel off the skin and chop the flesh.

2 Heat the olive oil in a large saucepan over low heat and fry the onion and garlic for 3–4 minutes until soft. Add the peppers and chillies, if using, and stir to combine.

3 Pour in the stock and beans, and bring to the boil. Simmer, covered, for 10 minutes. Process the soup in a blender or food processor, then pass it through a sieve. Cover and chill until required (or keep warm if serving hot).

4 To make the chilli cream, put the yogurt, chilli and basil into a food processor and pulse briefly to combine – leave some visible flakes of chilli and basil. Serve the soup topped with a spoonful of the chilli cream. (Store in the fridge for up to 3 days or freeze for 1 month.)

NUTRITIONAL INFORMATION PER SERVING
Protein 4.8g, **Carbohydrates** 13.6g of which sugars 6.5g, **Fat** 3.5g of which saturates 2.4g, **Kcals** 104

HEALTH BENEFITS
Cannellini beans provide protein as well as soluble fibre to support digestive health. Peppers are an excellent source of vitamin C and they also provide cancer-protective phytochemicals, such as lycopene and beta-carotene (the precursor for vitamin A).

Asian Turkey Patties with Dipping Sauce

The Asian flavours in these little patties make them especially tempting if your appetite is flat. The patties are rich in protein and B vitamins to perk up flagging energy levels, and the dipping sauce, made with yogurt, ginger and mint, can be helpful for settling digestive upsets. Serve with a mixed salad or steamed spring greens.

1 To make the sauce, put all the ingredients into a blender or food processor and blend briefly to combine. Chill until required.

2 Put the turkey into the blender or food processor with the fish sauce, tamari, ginger, onion and garlic. Blend to form a coarse purée. Transfer to a bowl, then cover and chill for 20 minutes.

3 With damp hands, shape the mixture into 8 patties. Heat the olive oil in a frying pan over medium heat and brown the patties in batches for 3–4 minutes on each side until cooked through. Serve the patties with the dipping sauce. (Store in the fridge for up to 3 days or freeze, uncooked, for 1 month.)

SERVES 2

PREPARATION TIME 15 minutes, plus chilling

COOKING TIME 16 minutes

250g/9oz skinless turkey breast, chopped
2 tbsp Thai fish sauce
1 tbsp tamari
1cm/½in piece fresh root ginger, peeled and grated
½ red onion, finely chopped
1 garlic clove, crushed
1 tbsp olive oil or coconut oil

Dipping sauce
200g/7oz/generous ¾ cup Greek yogurt or soya yogurt
2 green chillies, deseeded and chopped (optional)
1 large handful of mint leaves, finely chopped
1cm/½in piece fresh root ginger, peeled and grated
sea salt and freshly ground black pepper

NUTRITIONAL INFORMATION PER SERVING
Protein 36.6g, **Carbohydrates** 16.6g of which sugars 14.9g, **Fat** 2.2g of which saturates 1g, **Kcals** 225

HEALTH BENEFITS
Lean turkey meat is high in protein and is served here with ginger to aid digestion. The capsaicin in chillies gives them their characteristic pungency and it is a potent inhibitor of substance P, a neuropeptide associated with inflammatory processes. Studies also suggest that it may stop the spread of prostate cancer cells and lessen the expression of prostate-specific antigen (PSA).

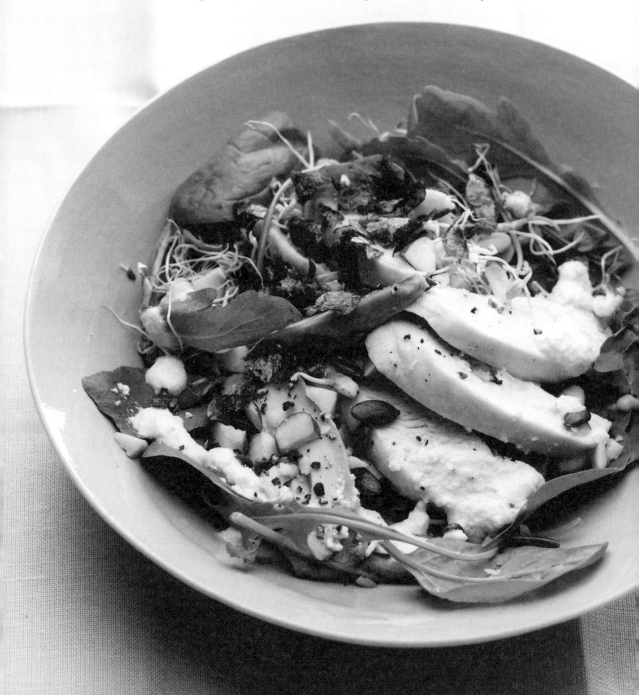

Super-Greens Salad with Chicken

A tangy and peppery, nutrient-dense green salad that is packed with vitamins, minerals, protein and healthy fats. The inclusion of nuts and seeds adds crunch and provides the essential minerals magnesium, manganese, iron, zinc and selenium. The roasted chicken, for additional protein, can be omitted or replaced with some tinned beans.

1 To make the dressing, soak the cashew nuts in water for 20 minutes, then drain. Put them into a blender or food processor with all the other dressing ingredients. Add 125ml/4fl oz/½ cup water, season lightly with pepper and process to make a light pouring consistency. Add a little more water if necessary.

2 In a large bowl, toss together the watercress, rocket, spinach, alfalfa and bean sprouts. Toss in a little of the dressing to just coat the leaves, if you like.

3 Slice the chicken. Serve the salad with the avocado slices, nuts, seeds and the chicken slices, and the nori sheet crumbled over the top. Drizzle over a little extra dressing. (Store, without dressing, in the fridge for up to 2 days.)

SERVES 4

PREPARATION TIME 10 minutes, plus 20 minutes soaking

115g/4oz each watercress, rocket leaves and baby spinach leaves
60g/2¼oz/1¾ cups alfalfa sprouts
60g/2¼oz mung bean sprouts
2 skinless roasted chicken breast fillets
1 ripe avocado, sliced
60g/2¼oz/heaped ⅓ cup Brazil nuts, roughly chopped
30g/1oz/¼ cup pumpkin seeds
1 nori sheet

Nut dressing
125g/4½oz/heaped ¾ cup cashew nuts
1 garlic clove
zest and juice of 1 lime
2 tsp spirulina or chlorella powder (optional)
2 tsp nutritional yeast flakes (optional)
freshly ground black pepper

NUTRITIONAL INFORMATION PER SERVING (WITH 1 TBSP DRESSING)
Protein 25.1g, **Carbohydrates** 4.2g of which sugars 1.5g, **Fat** 24.2g of which saturates 5.4g, **Kcal**s 335

HEALTH BENEFITS
Bitter leafy greens, such as rocket and watercress, are useful for stimulating digestive secretions and are packed with protective antioxidants. The use of the optional green superfood powders – spirulina and chlorella – in the dressing is an excellent way to add more amino acids (protein building blocks), vitamins and minerals to your diet.

Japanese Lamb Burgers with Wasabi Mayo

SERVES 4
PREPARATION TIME 15 minutes
COOKING TIME 15 minutes

400g/14oz lean minced lamb
1 garlic clove, crushed
1 red onion, grated
1 tbsp olive oil or coconut oil (optional)
sea salt and freshly ground black pepper

Wasabi mayonnaise
150g/5½oz silken tofu, cubed
3 tbsp olive oil or flaxseed oil
1 tbsp lemon juice
1 tsp xylitol or ½ tsp stevia
a pinch of matcha green tea powder
  (optional)
1 tsp wasabi powder

Quick-and-easy burgers accompanied by a tangy wasabi mayonnaise. The burgers can be frozen uncooked, making them ideal for cooking when you don't feel like preparing food. Either fry or grill them and serve with a green salad or steamed vegetables.

1 Put the lamb into a large bowl and add the garlic and onion. Season. Using your hands, mix well, then shape the mixture into 8 balls and press into burger shapes.

2 If frying the burgers, heat the oil in a frying pan over medium heat, fry the burgers for 5 minutes on each side or until cooked through. Alternatively, preheat the grill. Put the burgers on a foil-lined baking tray and grill for 6–7 minutes on each side until cooked through, but not over-browned.

3 To make the mayonnaise, put all the ingredients into a blender or food processor and process until smooth. Add a little water, if it seems too thick. Season the burgers lightly with pepper and serve with the mayonnaise. (The uncooked burgers can be frozen for up to 1 month.)

NUTRITIONAL INFORMATION PER SERVING
Protein 22.4g, **Carbohydrates** 2.7g of which sugars 2.2g, **Fat** 23.9g of which saturates 9.3g, **Kcals** 314

HEALTH BENEFITS
Lamb is grass fed, which is why it is a good source of omega-3 fats. It is also rich in protein, antioxidants, selenium and zinc for immune support, and B vitamins, which are important for energy. Distinctively flavoured Japanese wasabi is traditionally used for its flavour, but it is also included here for its anti-microbial, anti-cancer and anti-inflammatory benefits.

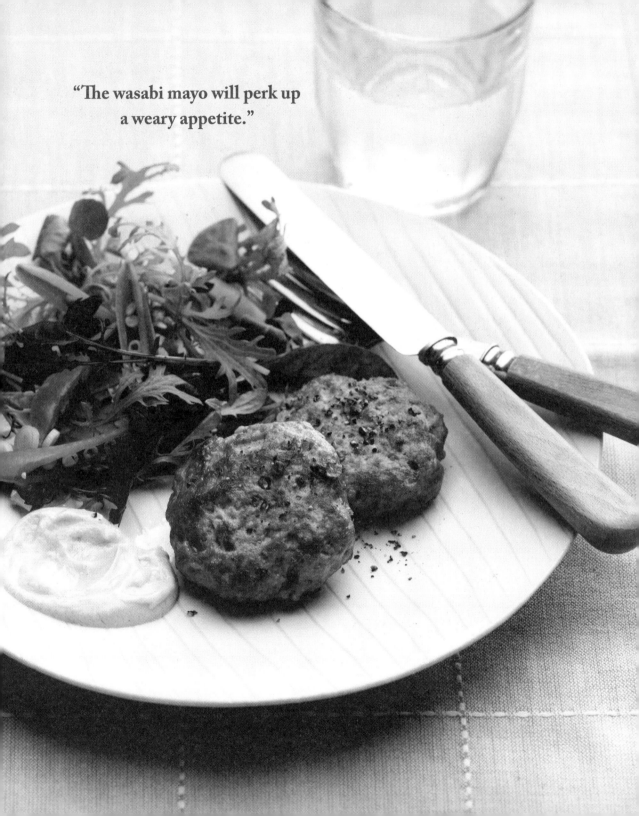

"The wasabi mayo will perk up a weary appetite."

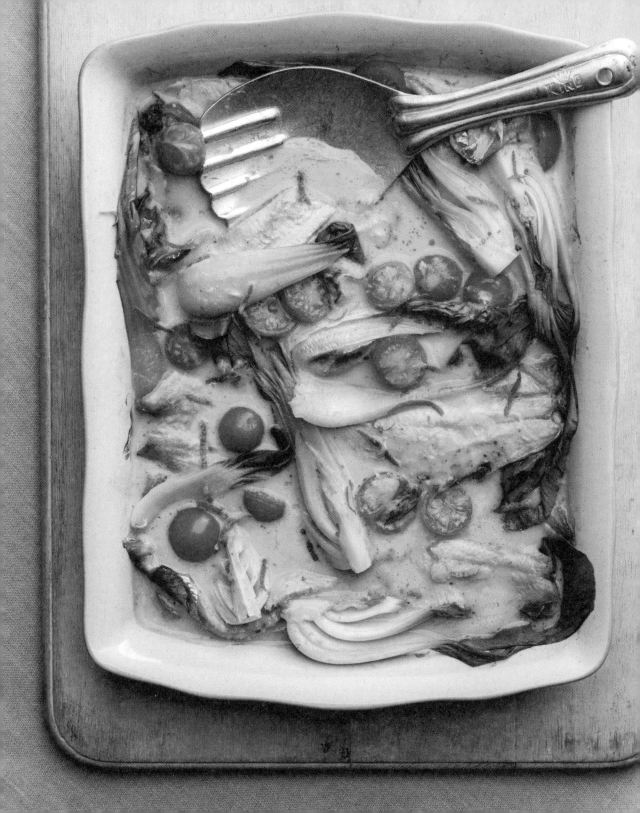

Coconut & Lime
Baked Sardines

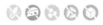

When you feel low in energy this dish will appeal, because it requires minimal preparation and is full of flavour. Sardines are cheap to buy and full of nutrients, and adding greens to the mix makes this a convenient one-pot meal that scores on all the healthy points. You can also make this with mackerel fillets.

1 Preheat the oven to 180°C/350°F/Gas 4. Mix a little of the coconut milk with the cornflour to form a smooth paste. In a saucepan, mix together the remaining coconut milk with the cornflour paste, curry paste, lime zest and juice, turmeric and stock, and warm gently, stirring continuously. Continue to stir until the mixture thickens. Season with salt and pepper.

2 Put the sardines, skin side down, in a large, shallow baking dish and add the pak choi. Pour over the coconut sauce and scatter the tomatoes between the sardines. Bake for 20 minutes or until the sardines are cooked through. Serve. (Best eaten fresh but can be stored in the fridge for up to 1 day.)

SERVES 4
PREPARATION TIME 10 minutes
COOKING TIME 25 minutes

400ml/14fl oz/generous 1½ cups tinned coconut milk
1 tbsp cornflour
2 tsp Thai red curry paste
zest and juice of 1 lime
1 tsp turmeric
80ml/2½fl oz/⅓ cup vegetable stock or water
8 sardines or 4 small mackerel, filleted
2 pak choi, cut into quarters
12 cherry tomatoes, cut in half
sea salt and freshly ground black pepper

NUTRITIONAL INFORMATION PER SERVING
Protein 43.5g, **Carbohydrates** 15.1g of which sugars 8.4g, **Fat** 20.2g of which saturates 5.7g, **Kcals** 413

HEALTH BENEFITS
Sardines are an abundant source of anti-inflammatory omega-3 fats, plus protein, to help maintain muscle mass and facilitate healing, as well as containing vitamin D, calcium and selenium.

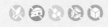

Sicilian Prawns

SERVES 4
PREPARATION TIME 15 minutes,
   plus 1 hour or overnight marinating
COOKING TIME 3 minutes

24 raw king prawns, peeled
1 tsp olive oil or coconut oil

Fresh herb dressing
2 tbsp capers, rinsed
1 tinned anchovy fillet
2 garlic cloves
a pinch of crushed chillies (optional)
1 handful each of mint leaves, coriander
   leaves and parsley leaves
3 tbsp balsamic vinegar
6 tbsp olive oil
sea salt and freshly ground black pepper

Roasted pepper salad
3 roasted red peppers from a jar, sliced
   into strips
1 red onion, finely chopped
2 tbsp capers, rinsed
8 pitted black olives, cut in half

Succulent king prawns marinated in a fresh herb dressing and served with a simple roasted pepper salad make this a quick-to-prepare meal that's rich in protein. Marinating the prawns in the dressing heightens their flavour. The salad and dressing can also be eaten without the prawns for a light and healthy meal or snack.

1 To make the dressing, put all the ingredients into a mini food processor and pulse to combine to a coarse texture.
2 Put the prawns into a shallow dish and pour over half the dressing. Cover and leave to marinate in the fridge for 1–2 hours or overnight.
3 Heat the olive oil in a frying pan over medium heat. Add the prawns with their dressing and cook for 2–3 minutes until cooked and pink.
4 Mix all the salad ingredients together in a bowl. Serve the salad topped with the prawns and with the remaining dressing drizzled over. (Store, without dressing, in the fridge for up to 2 days.)

NUTRITIONAL INFORMATION PER SERVING
Protein 12.8g, **Carbohydrates** 5.4g of which sugars 4.9g, **Fat** 25.6g of which saturates 4.3g, **Kcals** 306

HEALTH BENEFITS
Prawns are a good source of omega-3 fats, selenium and B vitamins. Docosahexaenoic acid (DHA), an omega-3 fatty acid found in prawns and cold-water fish, has been shown to reduce the size of tumours and enhance the positive effects of certain chemotherapy drugs while limiting their side effects.

Pan-Fried Squid with Red Cabbage & Walnuts

Serve this warm, crunchy salad as an alternative to coleslaw. Red cabbage is a nutrient-rich cruciferous vegetable and, combined with apple, nuts and cherries, makes a colourful and healthy dish. The salad is also nourishing served without the squid.

SERVES 4
PREPARATION TIME 10 minutes
COOKING TIME 10 minutes

60g/2¼oz/scant ½ cup walnut pieces
250g/9oz cleaned and prepared squid
2 tbsp olive oil or coconut oil
1 small red cabbage, shredded
2 garlic cloves, crushed
1cm/½in piece fresh root ginger, peeled and grated
½ red chilli, deseeded and finely diced (optional)
2 eating apples, grated
3 tbsp apple cider vinegar
2 tbsp tamari
1 tbsp fresh lime juice
2 tbsp chopped mint leaves
2 tbsp chopped coriander leaves
60g/2¼oz/½ cup dried unsweetened cherries
sea salt and freshly ground black pepper

1 Lightly toast the walnuts in a dry frying pan over medium heat for 1 minute, stirring, then chop them roughly. Set aside. Slit the squid tubes down one side, open them out, then score the inside lightly in a criss-cross pattern. Cut into bite-sized pieces. Season lightly with salt and pepper.

2 Heat the olive oil in a frying pan over medium heat. Add the squid tubes and tentacles and stir-fry for 1–2 minutes until just cooked. Remove with a slotted spoon and set aside. Add the cabbage, garlic, ginger and chilli, if using, and stir-fry for 3 minutes to soften the cabbage slightly.

3 Stir in the apples, vinegar, tamari and lime juice, and stir for 3–4 minutes until the cabbage is soft but still crunchy. Stir in the squid to warm through. Toss in the herbs and transfer to a bowl. Sprinkle over the walnuts and cherries, and season with salt and pepper. Serve immediately.

NUTRITIONAL INFORMATION PER SERVING
Protein 13.9g, **Carbohydrates** 22.9g of which sugars 21.6g, **Fat** 16.3g of which saturates 5.3g, **Kcals** 291

HEALTH BENEFITS
Seafood, such as squid, provides additional protein plus the minerals copper, selenium, phosphorus and magnesium. Selenium is particularly important for reducing inflammation. Copper is required by the body for the formation of red blood cells, which help to maintain energy levels.

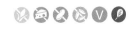

Hoisin Tempeh Skewers

SERVES 4

PREPARATION TIME 5 minutes,
plus at least 1 hour marinating

COOKING TIME 10 minutes

400g/14oz tempeh

3 tbsp hoisin sauce

2 tbsp tamari

2cm/¾in piece fresh root ginger, peeled
and grated

1 red chilli, deseeded and chopped
(optional)

1 garlic clove, crushed

3 tbsp mirin or 1 tbsp rice wine

2 tbsp vegetable stock or water

Pickled cucumber salad

½ cucumber

1 small red chilli, deseeded and thinly
sliced into ribbons (optional)

juice of ½ lime

2 tbsp rice wine vinegar

2 tbsp tamari

1 tbsp toasted nori flakes

2 tbsp finely chopped coriander, to serve

Nutty-tasting tempeh is a highly nutritious fermented food made from soya beans. It is rich in protein and fibre, and makes a sustaining and energizing light dish that is also suitable for snacking on. It is served here with a pickled cucumber salad.

1 Pat the tempeh dry and cut it into 2cm/¾in cubes. Mix together the hoisin sauce, tamari, ginger, chilli, if using, garlic, mirin and stock. Put the tempeh into a shallow dish and pour over the marinade. Leave to marinate for 1 hour or overnight.

2 To make the salad, cut the cucumber into long ribbons using a vegetable peeler. Put them into a bowl with the chilli, if using. Mix together the remaining ingredients and pour over the cucumber. Leave to marinate for 30 minutes. Meanwhile, soak 8 wooden skewers in water.

3 Preheat the grill to high. Line a baking tray with baking parchment. Thread 4 pieces of tempeh on to each skewer and put on to the tray. Grill for 8–10 minutes until golden, turning occasionally and brushing with marinade. Sprinkle coriander over the salad and serve with the tempeh. (Store in the fridge for up to 2 days.)

NUTRITIONAL INFORMATION PER SERVING
Protein 21.7g, **Carbohydrates** 12.5g of which sugars 2.1g, **Fat** 6.9g of which saturates 0g, **Kcals** 210

HEALTH BENEFITS
Tempeh is rich in fibre, antioxidants and naturally occurring isoflavones, including genistein, which has been linked to a lower incidence of certain cancers such as prostate. Genistein has been shown to induce the chemicals that block cell cycling, thus preventing the proliferation of cancerous cells in the prostate.

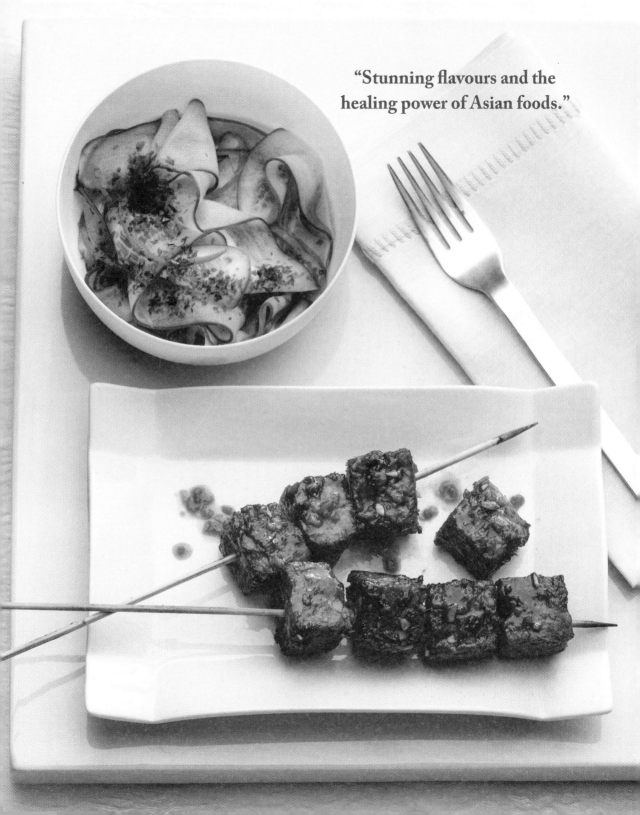

"Stunning flavours and the healing power of Asian foods."

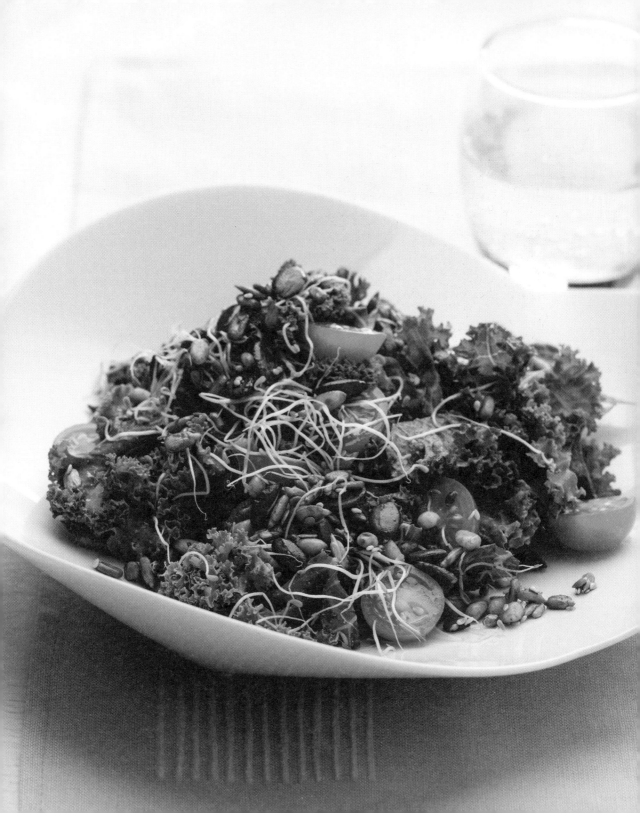

Wilted Kale Salad with Toasted Seeds

This simple, cleansing salad is quick to prepare and ideal for a very light lunch to accompany hard-boiled eggs or some feta cheese. The toasted seeds and nuts can also be eaten as a tasty and wholesome snack, so it's worth making up a batch and keeping it in an airtight container ready to eat with a fruit juice or smoothie.

1 To make the toasted seeds and nuts, put them in a dry frying pan over medium heat and lightly toast for 1 minute, stirring. As they begin to colour, pour over the tamari and stir to combine. Stir for 1–2 minutes until crisp. Leave to cool.

2 Put the kale into a large bowl and sprinkle over the garlic salt and yeast flakes, if using. Massage with your hands to allow the kale to soften. Put the avocado, lemon juice, cumin, oil and tamari into a blender or food processor and process until smooth. Mix into the kale so that it is thoroughly coated. Stir in the tomatoes and sprinkle over the alfalfa sprouts and toasted seeds and nuts, then serve. (Store in the fridge for up to 2 days.)

SERVES 4
PREPARATION TIME 10 minutes
COOKING TIME 3 minutes

250g/9oz kale, large stems discarded, leaves roughly chopped
1 tsp garlic salt
1 tbsp nutritional yeast flakes (optional)
1 ripe avocado, pitted and peeled
3 tbsp lemon juice
½ tsp ground cumin
1 tbsp olive oil or flaxseed oil
2 tsp tamari
200g/7oz/1⅓ cups cherry tomatoes, cut in half
1 handful of alfalfa sprouts

Toasted seeds and nuts

2 tbsp pine nuts
6 tbsp mixed seeds, such as sunflower seeds, pumpkin seeds and hemp seeds
2 tbsp tamari

NUTRITIONAL INFORMATION PER SERVING
Protein 9.8g, **Carbohydrates** 7.8g of which sugars 4.8g, **Fat** 24.3g of which saturates 3.1g, **Kcals** 289

HEALTH BENEFITS
Kale is a cruciferous super-food rich in glucosinolates, which can play a primary role in protection against many forms of cancer. It is also packed with flavonoids: antioxidants that help lower inflammation and protect against cell damage. (People with thyroid problems should limit their intake of raw cruciferous vegetables, because they can lower the function of the thyroid and reduce metabolism.)

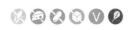

Celeriac, Apple & Fennel Remoulade

SERVES 4
PREPARATION TIME 15 minutes

½ celeriac
2 apples, cored and cut
  into thin slices
2 fennel bulbs, cut into thin slices
2 tbsp capers, rinsed and finely chopped
8 small gherkins, finely chopped
3 tbsp chopped parsley leaves, plus extra
  to serve
2 tbsp chopped mint leaves
sea salt and freshly ground black pepper

Tofu mayonnaise
150g/5½oz silken tofu
1 tbsp Dijon mustard
zest and juice of 1 lemon
150ml/5fl oz/scant ⅔ cup olive oil or
  omega blended oil (a combination of
  flaxseed oil, olive oil, hempseed oil)
a little vegetable stock or water, if needed

This dish is dairy-free, and the tofu mayonnaise provides protein, calcium, magnesium and phytoestrogens. To add a little colour and additional liver support, try including some grated raw beetroot. For some extra protein, add a few walnuts or pecan nuts, or serve the salad with meat or fish. Silken tofu, used for the dressing, is a soft tofu suitable for making into sauces and desserts.

1 To make the mayonnaise, put the tofu, mustard and lemon juice into a blender or food processor and switch on. Add the oil in a steady stream to form a thick, creamy sauce. You may need to add a little water or stock to thin it slightly. Stir in the lemon zest and set aside.
2 Cut the celeriac into matchstick strips and put into a large bowl with the apples and fennel. Add the capers, gherkins, parsley and mint. Pour over the tofu mayonnaise and mix to combine. Season with salt and pepper, and sprinkle with parsley, then serve. (Store in the fridge for up to 3 days.)

NUTRITIONAL INFORMATION PER SERVING
Protein 4.9g, **Carbohydrates** 6.9g of which sugars 6.5g, **Fat** 37.1g of which saturates 3.5g, **Kcals** 407

HEALTH BENEFITS
Fennel is well known for its digestive properties and aids fat digestion by stimulating the gall bladder and increasing the flow of bile. Apples are a good source of pectin – a soluble fibre that assists digestion.

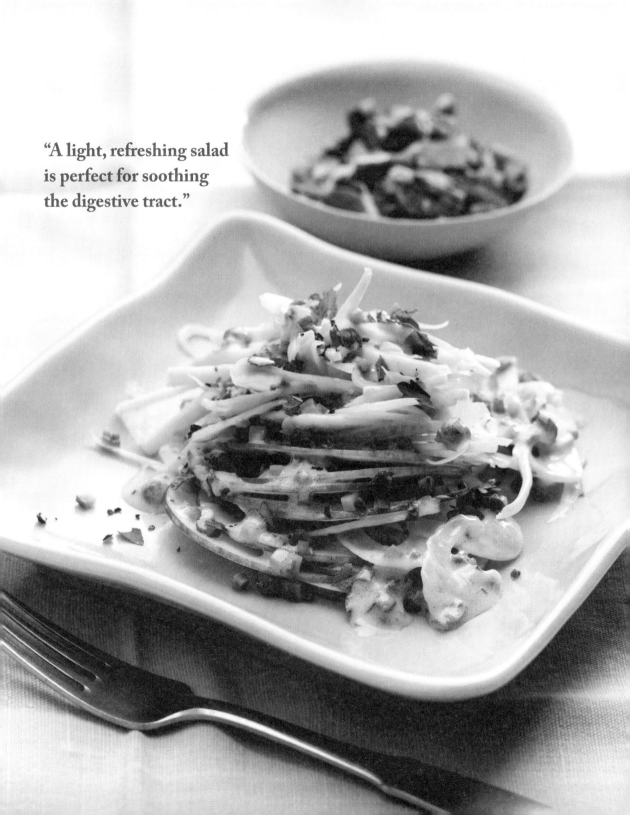

"A light, refreshing salad is perfect for soothing the digestive tract."

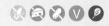

SERVES 4

PREPARATION TIME 10 minutes,
    plus 15 minutes soaking

COOKING TIME 5 minutes

60g/2¼oz mixed dried seaweed

150g/5½oz/2 cups frozen edamame
    (soya beans)

1 cucumber

200g/7oz rocket leaves or a mixture of
    leafy greens

3 spring onions, thinly sliced

Lime soy dressing

2 tbsp olive oil or flaxseed oil

1cm/½in piece fresh root ginger, peeled
    and grated

zest and juice of 1 lime

1 tbsp tamari

Mixed Sea Vegetable & Cucumber Salad

Adding sea vegetables to salad is an easy way to increase your intake of iodine, which is typically low in many people's diets and a deficiency has been linked to the development of breast cancer. This Japanese-inspired dish is light and refreshing and can be served with steamed fish or prawns.

1 Soak the seaweed in water for 15 minutes or according to the packet instructions, then drain thoroughly. Put the edamame in a steamer and steam over high heat for 5 minutes or until just tender, then drain and refresh under cold water.

2 Cut the cucumber into long strips using a vegetable peeler. Put all the dressing ingredients into a small bowl and whisk well.

3 Toss the rocket, sea vegetables, spring onions, cucumber and edamame together in a large bowl, then drizzle over the dressing and toss to coat before serving. (Store, without dressing, in the fridge for up to 2 days.)

NUTRITIONAL INFORMATION PER SERVING
Protein 11.9g, **Carbohydrates** 4.3g of which sugars 3.2g, **Fat** 10.5g of which saturates 1.2g, **Kcals** 163

HEALTH BENEFITS
Sea vegetables such as dulse, kelp, nori and arame are rich in trace minerals and sulphur, which may play a role in lowering the risk of oestrogen-related cancers, including breast cancer.

Warm Lentil & Bean Salad

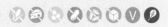

Cannellini beans are creamy in texture and contrast beautifully with the crunchy celery and Puy lentils, and the sweet flavour of roasted tomatoes. You can use tinned Puy lentils, if you prefer, for this sustaining salad.

1 Preheat the oven to 200°C/400°F/Gas 6. Mix together 2 tablespoons of the olive oil and all the garlic. Put the cherry tomatoes in a baking dish and drizzle over the garlic oil. Roast for 10 minutes or until just softened.

2 Meanwhile, put the lentils in a saucepan and add enough water to cover them. Bring to the boil, then simmer for 10–12 minutes until just cooked. Drain and rinse.

3 Heat the remaining olive oil in a frying pan over medium heat and gently fry the onion and celery for 2–3 minutes until soft. Add the lentils, beans and balsamic vinegar, and cook for 1–2 minutes to heat through. Toss in the tomatoes and herbs, and season with salt and pepper. Serve. (Store in the fridge for up to 3 days.)

SERVES 4
PREPARATION TIME 10 minutes
COOKING TIME 20 minutes

3 tbsp olive oil
3 garlic cloves, crushed
250g/9oz/heaped 1¾ cups cherry tomatoes, cut in half
200g/7oz/1 cup Puy lentils, rinsed
1 red onion, finely chopped
1 celery stick, finely chopped
400g/14oz/2 cups tinned cannellini beans, drained and rinsed
2 tbsp balsamic vinegar
2 tbsp finely chopped mint leaves
2 tbsp finely chopped parsley leaves
sea salt and freshly ground black pepper

NUTRITIONAL INFORMATION PER SERVING
Protein 16.6g, **Carbohydrates** 34.3g of which sugars 5.1g, **Fat** 8.3g of which saturates 2.8g, **Kcals** 281

HEALTH BENEFITS
Roasting the tomatoes optimizes the availability of lycopene: a potent antioxidant for helping with cancer recovery. Beans and lentils are a good source of protein, soluble fibre and phytoestrogens, and the garlic has anti-inflammatory properties.

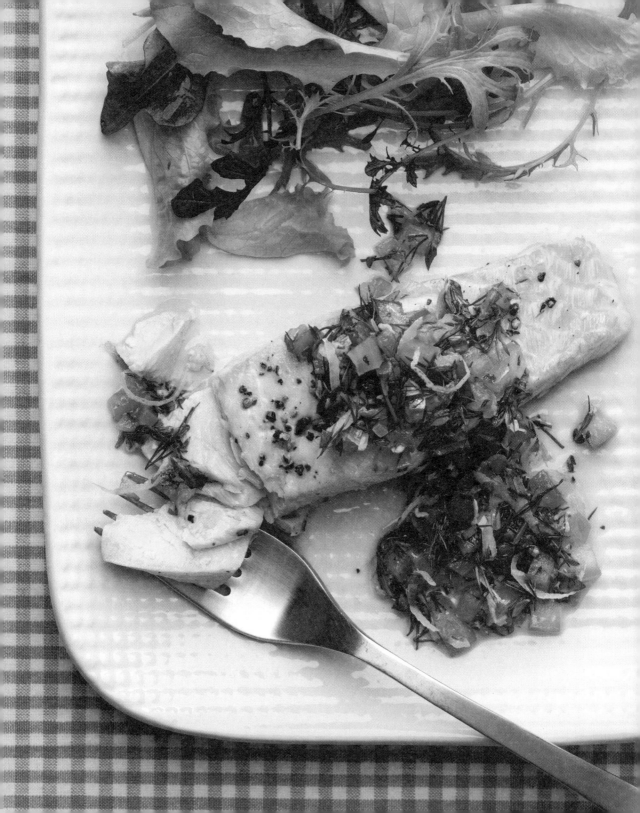

Main Meals

During cancer treatment and recovery there may be times when you crave warming comfort foods that are rich in flavour and also full of nourishing ingredients. In this chapter we have created a selection of appealing, easy-to-assemble main meals to satisfy your appetite while also optimizing nutrition.

We focus on using key ingredients to help protect and heal the body, while ensuring that each meal is tempting in flavour and appearance. There are new slants on favourites, such as our Mixed Seafood Pie and Turkey & Pistachio Korma, plus the classic Venison with Zesty Gremolata, and more exotic combinations such as Ginger & Umeboshi Chicken and our Tamarind-Spiced Mackerel. Many of the dishes are suitable for storing, freezing or preparing in advance.

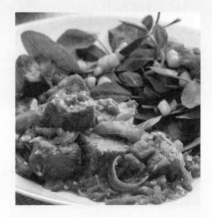

Opposite: Salmon with Sauce Vierge (page 104)
Above: Roasted Tempeh with Piperade Sauce (page 110)

SERVES 4
PREPARATION TIME 10 minutes
COOKING TIME 10 minutes

60g/2¼oz/heaped ⅓ cup cashew nuts
1 egg
1 tbsp cornflour
450g/1lb skinless chicken breast fillets,
    sliced
1 tbsp olive oil or coconut oil
4 spring onions, sliced
100g/3½oz mangetout, trimmed
1 pak choi, leaves separated
1 yellow pepper, deseeded and sliced
    into strips
1 red pepper, deseeded and sliced
    into strips
150g/5½oz shiitake mushrooms, sliced
4 tbsp chicken stock
juice of 1 lime
2–3 tbsp tamari
2 tbsp coriander leaves
sea salt and freshly ground black pepper

Chicken & Cashew Nut Stir-Fry

For this super-quick dish, strips of chicken flavoured with coriander and lime are tossed with a colourful medley of vegetables and toasted nuts. Choose organic chicken if possible to reduce your exposure to added hormones and antibiotics. Serve with buckwheat or wholewheat noodles.

1 Lightly toast the nuts in a dry frying pan over medium heat for 1 minute, stirring, and set aside. Put the egg into a large bowl, add the cornflour and a pinch of salt, and whisk to combine. Add the chicken and coat with the egg mixture.

2 Heat a frying pan or wok with the olive oil over medium heat. Stir-fry the chicken for 4–5 minutes until golden, then remove with a slotted spoon.

3 Add the spring onions and stir-fry for a few seconds. Add the mangetout, pak choi and peppers, and stir-fry for 1 minute or until just softened. Add the chicken, mushrooms, stock, lime juice and tamari to taste. Simmer for 1 minute or until the mushrooms have softened. Stir in the nuts and coriander, then season with salt and pepper. Serve. (Store in the fridge for up to 3 days.)

NUTRITIONAL INFORMATION PER SERVING
Protein 34.9g, **Carbohydrates** 17g of which sugars 8.2g, **Fat** 12.9g of which saturates 4.2g, **Kcals** 323

HEALTH BENEFITS
Chicken is an energizing food, rich in B vitamins and protein and low in saturated fats. It is an excellent source of the cancer-protective B vitamin, niacin, which helps to protect components of DNA.

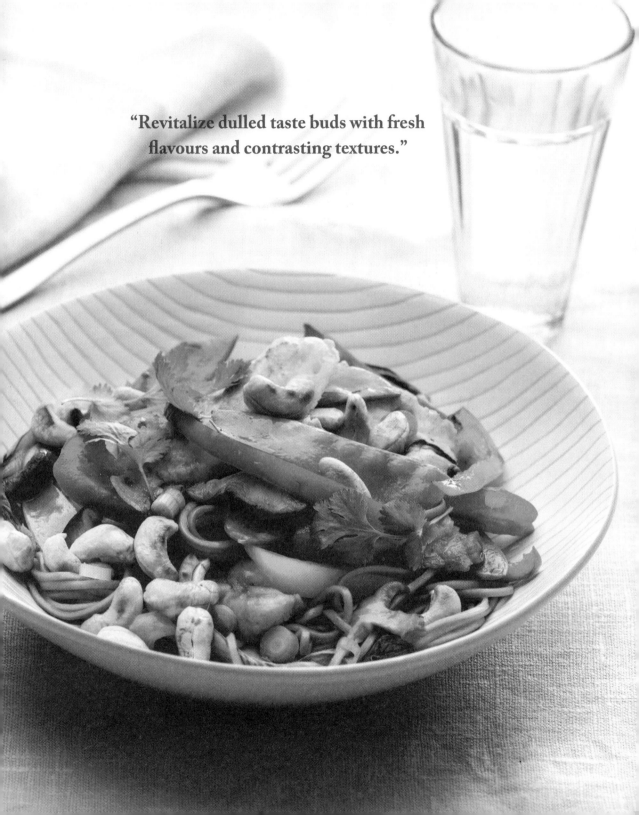

"Revitalize dulled taste buds with fresh flavours and contrasting textures."

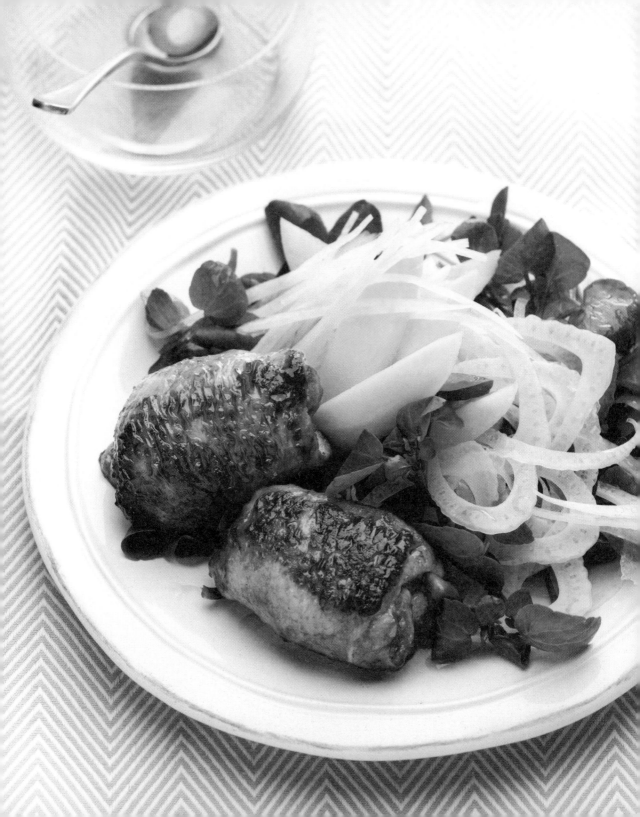

Ginger & Umeboshi Chicken

Umeboshi paste is a traditional Japanese condiment that has a fruity, sour and tangy flavour. It is combined here with ginger and honey to create a sticky glaze for chicken. The dish is served with a digestion-supporting salad of watercress, fennel and white radish.

1 Put the chicken in a shallow dish. Mix together the honey, umeboshi paste and spices. Pour the mixture over the chicken and leave to marinate for 15 minutes.

2 Heat the olive oil in a frying pan over medium heat, add the chicken thighs and cook gently for 3–4 minutes until browned all over. Pour in the remaining marinade and the chicken stock. Cover the pan and cook gently for 6–7 minutes until the thighs are cooked through.

3 Toss the watercress, mango, daikon, fennel, lemon juice and oil lightly together in a bowl (or arrange the salad on the plates and drizzle with the lemon and oil). Top with the chicken to serve. (Leftovers can be stored in the fridge for up to 2 days.)

SERVES 4

PREPARATION TIME 10 minutes, plus 15 minutes marinating

COOKING TIME 10 minutes

8 boneless chicken thighs, with skin
3 tbsp raw honey
1 tbsp umeboshi paste/plum paste
5mm/¼in piece fresh root ginger, peeled and grated
½ tsp Chinese five-spice powder
a pinch of paprika
1 tbsp olive oil or coconut oil
4 tbsp chicken or vegetable stock
60g/2¼oz watercress
1 small ripe mango, peeled, pitted and sliced
115g/4oz daikon or white radish, or kohlrabi, cut into matchstick strips
1 fennel bulb, thinly sliced
1 tbsp lemon juice
1 tbsp olive oil or flaxseed oil

NUTRITIONAL INFORMATION PER SERVING

Protein 27.3g, **Carbohydrates** 19.6g of which sugars 19.6g, **Fat** 15g of which saturates 4.8g, **Kcals** 324

HEALTH BENEFITS

Umeboshi, made from Japanese pickled plum, is traditionally used in Japanese dishes to stimulate the digestion. The plums are also known for their health-giving alkalizing properties – an alkaline environment is thought to reduce the risk of cancer.

Turkey & Pistachio Korma

SERVES 4

PREPARATION TIME 15 minutes,
 plus 30 minutes marinating

COOKING TIME 30 minutes

400g/14oz skinless turkey breast, sliced

3 tbsp Greek or soya yogurt

½ tsp garam masala

5mm/¼in piece fresh root ginger, grated

½ green chilli, deseeded and finely
 chopped (optional)

½ tsp turmeric

1 tsp tamarind paste

1 garlic clove, crushed

Nut sauce

2 onions, finely chopped

1cm/½in piece of fresh root ginger, grated

½ tsp turmeric

2 garlic cloves, crushed

60g/2¼oz/heaped ⅓ cup pistachio nuts

1 tbsp olive oil or coconut oil

200ml/7fl oz/scant 1 cup chicken stock

150g/5½oz/scant ⅔ cup Greek or soya
 yogurt

200g/7oz baby spinach leaves

2 tbsp chopped coriander leaves, plus
 extra leaves to serve

Pistachio nuts create a rich sauce in this well-rounded curry. The addition of the spiced yogurt marinade keeps the turkey moist and tender, and tamarind gives it a tangy edge. For a dairy-free option you could use soya or coconut yogurt instead of the Greek yogurt. Serve with steamed vegetables and a little brown rice.

1 Put the turkey in a shallow dish. Mix the remaining ingredients together and rub into the turkey. Leave to marinate for 30 minutes.

2 To make the nut sauce, put the onions, spices and garlic into a blender or food processor and pulse to make a paste. Lightly toast the nuts in a dry frying pan over medium heat for 1 minute. Set the nuts aside. Add the olive oil to the pan and heat. Add the turkey and marinade, and cook for 2–3 minutes to brown the turkey. Add the paste and stir for 2 minutes, then pour in the stock. Bring to the boil and simmer for 15 minutes or until the turkey is cooked.

3 Put the nuts and yogurt into a blender or food processor and process until smooth. Add the yogurt sauce to the pan with the spinach and coriander, bring to the boil and simmer for 5 minutes or until the spinach has wilted. Serve sprinkled with extra coriander leaves. (Store in the fridge for up to 3 days.)

NUTRITIONAL INFORMATION PER SERVING

Protein 33.2g, **Carbohydrates** 14.1g of which sugars 10.4g, **Fat** 12.4g of which saturates 4g, **Kcals** 301

HEALTH BENEFITS

Turkey is an excellent source of protein, useful for supporting muscle mass and preventing cachexia (weight loss) in cancer patients.

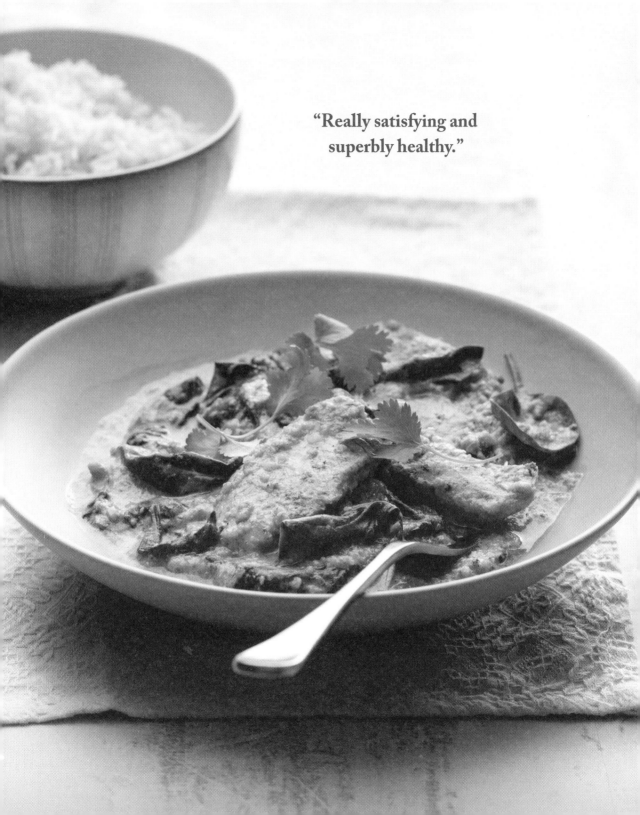

"Really satisfying and superbly healthy."

Balsamic Braised Duck

SERVES 4

PREPARATION TIME 15 minutes,
   plus 30 minutes marinating

COOKING TIME 20 minutes

4 skinless, boneless duck breasts
1 tbsp plus 150ml/5fl oz/scant ⅔ cup
   balsamic vinegar
2 tsp raw honey
2 tbsp tamari
30g/1oz/scant 1 cup dried shiitake
   mushrooms
1 tbsp olive oil or coconut oil
2 onions, finely chopped
2 garlic cloves, crushed
200g/7oz mixed mushrooms, including
   shiitake, sliced
250ml/9fl oz/1 cup chicken stock
1 tbsp cornflour
1 tbsp cranberry or redcurrant jelly
1 handful of parsley, leaves chopped
sea salt and freshly ground black pepper

Shiitake mushrooms add an intense flavour to this tangy sauce to accompany duck breasts. This attractive dish will tempt you to eat well when you may feel disinclined to prepare food. Serve with sweet potatoes and a salad.

1 Put the duck breasts in a shallow dish. Mix together the 1 tablespoon balsamic vinegar, the honey and tamari, and pour it over the duck. Leave to marinate for 30 minutes. Soak the mushrooms in boiling water to cover for 15 minutes, then drain and reserve the liquid. Chop the mushrooms. Preheat the oven to 190°C/375°F/Gas 5.

2 Heat an ovenproof frying pan over medium heat and brown the duck on each side. Put into the oven for 12–15 minutes until cooked through. Leave to rest, then slice thinly.

3 Meanwhile, put the olive oil in the frying pan and gently fry the onions and garlic for 2–3 minutes until soft. Add all the mushrooms, and stir for 1 minute. Pour in the remaining vinegar, the stock and reserved mushroom liquid. Bring to the boil, then simmer for 5 minutes. Mix the cornflour with 2 tablespoons water, then add to the pan and stir to thicken. Add the duck, cranberry jelly and parsley, then season and serve. (Store leftovers in the fridge for up to 2 days.)

NUTRITIONAL INFORMATION PER SERVING
Protein 23.3g, **Carbohydrates** 14.4g of which sugars 7.1g, **Fat** 9.8g of which saturates 4.1g, **Kcals** 246

HEALTH BENEFITS
Shiitake mushrooms have immune-boosting and cancer-protective properties, largely due to the presence of polysaccharides and polysaccharide glucans, which stimulate immune response and help macrophage cells in clearing potentially cancerous cells. They are also a source of vitamin D2, the B vitamins and the minerals manganese, phosphorus, potassium, selenium, copper and zinc.

Venison with Zesty Gremolata

Succulent and flavoursome venison is a good source
of protein yet it is low in saturated fat. It benefits from
long, slow cooking, and here it is braised with vegetables
and olives to increase the depth of flavour. The orange
segments and gremolata contrast well with the richness of
the meat. Serve with steamed broccoli.

1 Preheat the oven to 180°C/350°F/Gas 4. Heat 1 tablespoon
of the olive oil in a heavy-based flameproof casserole over
medium heat and gently fry the onion, celery, carrot and
garlic for 4–5 minutes until lightly golden. Remove from
the pan and set aside.

2 Put the venison into a plastic bag with the flour and some
salt and pepper, and shake to coat. Add a little more olive
oil to the pan, if needed, then fry the venison in batches,
stirring, until lightly browned.

3 Return the onion mixture to the pan, then add the wine,
tomatoes, stock and olives. Bring to the boil, then cover
and cook in the oven for 1½ hours or until tender.

4 Remove from the oven and check the seasoning. Stir in the
orange segments. Mix together the zests with the parsley
and scatter over the casserole. Serve. (Store leftovers in the
fridge for up to 2 days.)

SERVES 4

PREPARATION TIME 15 minutes

COOKING TIME 1 hour 45 minutes

1–2 tbsp olive oil or coconut oil

1 onion, finely chopped

2 celery sticks, chopped

1 carrot, diced

2 garlic cloves, chopped

600g/1lb 5oz venison shoulder or
boneless leg, cut into large chunks

3 tbsp wholemeal plain flour or rice flour

250ml/9fl oz/1 cup red wine, or lamb or
beef stock

400g/14oz/scant 1⅔ cups tinned chopped
tomatoes

500ml/17fl oz/2 cups lamb or beef stock

200g/7oz/1⅔ cups pitted green olives

2 oranges, in segments or thinly sliced

zest of 2 oranges

zest of 1 lemon

2 tbsp finely chopped parsley leaves

sea salt and freshly ground black pepper

NUTRITIONAL INFORMATION PER SERVING

Protein 36.9g, **Carbohydrates** 18.5g of which sugars 9.7g, **Fat** 10.7g of which saturates 4.1g, **Kcals** 361

HEALTH BENEFITS

Venison contains energizing iron and B vitamins as well as zinc and selenium for immune and antioxidant support.

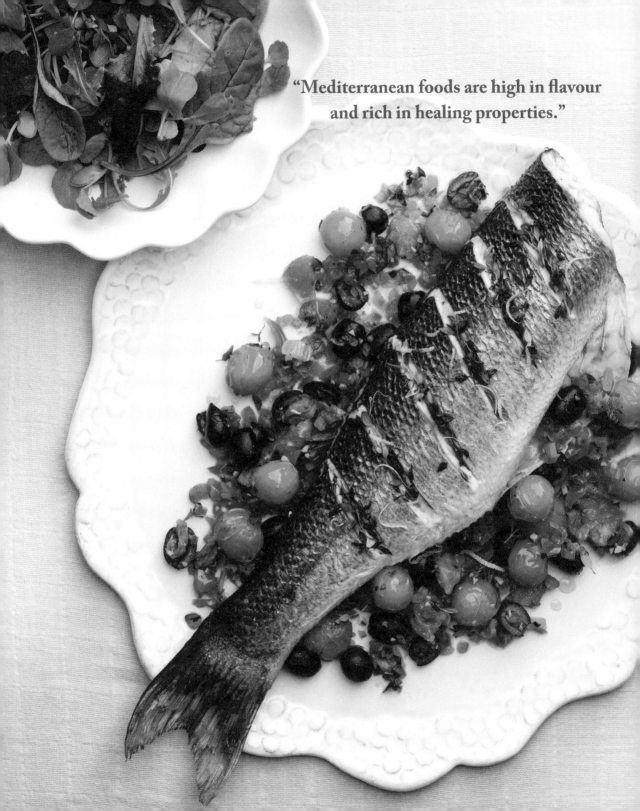

"Mediterranean foods are high in flavour and rich in healing properties."

Baked Sea Bass with Olives & Tomatoes

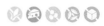

Baking sea bass on a bed of Mediterranean vegetables makes it beautifully moist and full of flavour. It's simple to prepare, taking only 15 minutes, and is packed with antioxidant-rich and anti-inflammatory ingredients. Serve with salad, or steamed shredded kale or spinach.

SERVES 4

PREPARATION TIME 15 minutes

COOKING TIME 30 minutes

½ tsp coriander seeds

1 tbsp olive oil or coconut oil

1 red onion, roughly chopped

2 garlic cloves, crushed

leaves from 3 thyme sprigs, plus
   1 small bunch of fresh thyme sprigs

115g/4oz/scant 1 cup pitted black olives,
   roughly chopped

60g/2¼oz/heaped ⅓ cup sun-dried
   tomatoes in oil, drained and roughly
   chopped

16 cherry tomatoes

1 large sea bass or trout, head removed,
   scaled and gutted

zest of 1 lemon

olive oil, for drizzling

sea salt and freshly ground black pepper

1 Preheat the oven to 190°C/375°F/Gas 5. Toast the coriander seeds in a dry frying pan over medium heat for 1 minute, then crush using a mortar and pestle. Heat the olive oil in the frying pan over medium heat. Add the onion, coriander and garlic, and fry gently for 2–3 minutes until the onion starts to soften. Stir in the thyme leaves, olives and the sun-dried and cherry tomatoes.

2 Season with salt and pepper, then transfer to a large, shallow ovenproof dish. Using a sharp knife, slash the skin of the fish diagonally along each side. Push sprigs of thyme into the cuts. Sprinkle over the lemon zest, then put the fish on top of the tomato mixture.

3 Drizzle over a little olive oil and cook in the oven for 20–25 minutes until the fish is cooked through. Serve. (Store leftovers in the fridge for up to 1 day.)

NUTRITIONAL INFORMATION PER SERVING

Protein 30.5g, **Carbohydrates** 3.4g of which sugars 2.7g, **Fat** 21.1g of which saturates 4.6g, **Kcals** 323

HEALTH BENEFITS

Sea bass is a good source of omega-3 fats and also provides B vitamins, magnesium and the antioxidant mineral selenium.

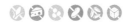

Salmon with Sauce Vierge

SERVES 4

PREPARATION TIME 10 minutes

COOKING TIME 10 minutes,
  plus 10 minutes infusing

125ml/4fl oz/½ cup, plus 1 tbsp olive oil
zest and juice of 1 lemon
2 tomatoes, deseeded and finely diced
1 shallot, finely chopped
2 garlic cloves, crushed
3 tbsp chopped tarragon leaves
2 tbsp chopped dill leaves
2 tbsp chopped parsley leaves
2 tbsp chopped chervil leaves
4 salmon fillets (about 600g/1lb 5oz total
  weight), with skin
sea salt and freshly ground black pepper

A superbly healthy and flavourful dish. The light, herb
sauce gives a fresh dimension to rich-tasting salmon.
This dish is straightforward to prepare and can be made
ahead and chilled until needed. Try to use wild salmon in
preference to farmed. Serve with a salad of mixed leaves.

1 Pour the 125ml/4fl oz/½ cup olive oil into a small
   saucepan. Stir in the lemon zest and juice, then add the
   tomatoes, shallot and garlic. Heat the sauce very gently
   until just warm. Turn off the heat and add the herbs.
   Season with salt and pepper, then leave to infuse for
   10 minutes.

2 Season the salmon with black pepper to taste. Heat the
   1 tablespoon olive oil in a frying pan over medium heat.
   Add the salmon, skin side down, and fry for 2–3 minutes
   until the skin is golden brown.

3 Turn the fillets over and cook for a further 2–3 minutes,
   until the fish is cooked through. Pour the herb sauce into
   the frying pan and warm through. Serve the salmon with
   the sauce spooned over.

NUTRITIONAL INFORMATION PER SERVING

Protein 23.3g, **Carbohydrates** 1.3g of which sugars 0.9g, **Fat** 46g of which saturates 8.6g, **Kcals** 512

HEALTH BENEFITS

Salmon is high in protein and rich in omega-3 essential fatty acids. Fresh herbs contain antioxidants and volatile oils that possess cancer-
protective properties.

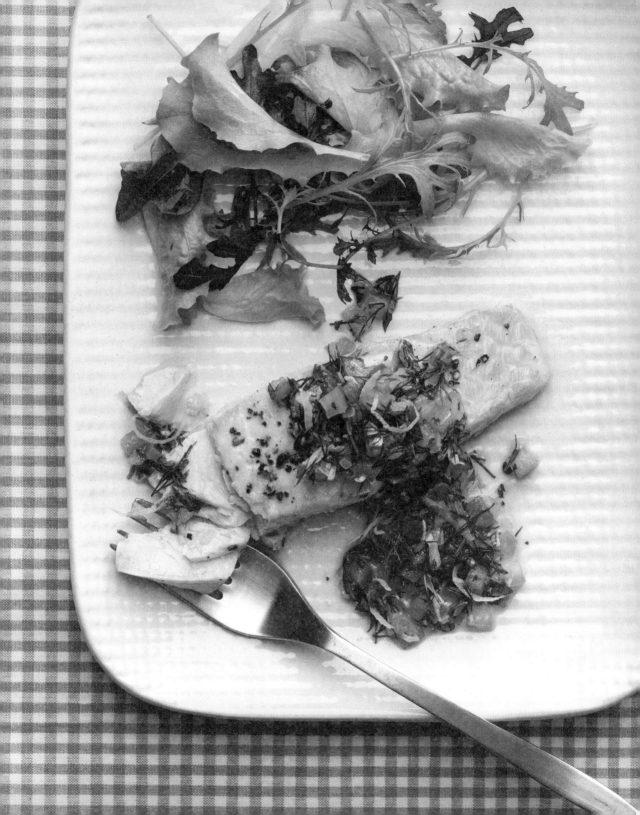

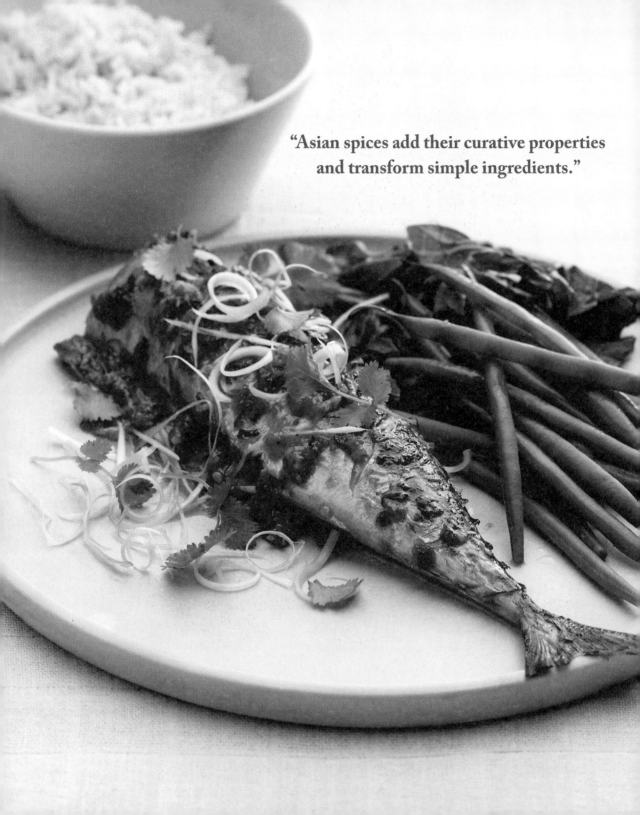

"Asian spices add their curative properties and transform simple ingredients."

Tamarind-Spiced Mackerel

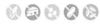

The rich, oily texture of mackerel contrasts well with the tangy, sour flavour of the tamarind in this Asian-inspired dish that is fragrant with lemongrass, ginger and mint. Oily fish is filling and sustaining as well as being rich in omega-3 essential fats. Serve with brown rice, green beans and steamed sliced spring greens.

1 In a small bowl, mix together the tamarind, lemongrass, chilli powder, if using, ginger, honey and mint.
2 Preheat the grill. Using a sharp knife, slash the skin of the mackerel on either side. Put the mackerel into a shallow ovenproof dish and pour over the tamarind sauce. Coat thoroughly on both sides.
3 Put the dish under the grill and cook for 10 minutes or until cooked through. Serve sprinkled with coriander and spring onions. (Leftovers can be stored in the fridge for up to 1 day.)

SERVES 4
PREPARATION TIME 10 minutes
COOKING TIME 10 minutes

60g/2¼oz/¼ cup tamarind paste
1 lemongrass stalk, tough parts removed, finely chopped
1 tsp chilli powder (optional)
1cm/½in piece fresh root ginger, peeled and grated
2 tbsp raw honey
1 small bunch of mint, leaves chopped
4 mackerel, head removed and cleaned
1 small handful of coriander leaves
2 spring onions, finely sliced

NUTRITIONAL INFORMATION PER SERVING
Protein 38g, **Carbohydrates** 13.1g of which sugars 4.9g, **Fat** 32.4g of which saturates 6.6g, **Kcals** 490

HEALTH BENEFITS
Tamarind is rich in soluble fibre, important for supporting bowel health and stabilizing blood sugar levels. It also contains antioxidants and phytochemicals, including limonene, known for its anti-cancer properties.

Miso-Glazed Salmon

SERVES 4
PREPARATION TIME 10 minutes,
    plus overnight marinating
COOKING TIME 25 minutes

600g/1lb 5oz salmon fillet, with skin, or
    4 boneless salmon fillets (about 150g/
    5½oz each)
4 tbsp Chinese rice wine
2 tbsp mirin or 1 tbsp rice wine
4 tbsp white miso paste
1 tbsp tamari
1 tbsp xylitol or a pinch of stevia
    (optional)
1 handful of coriander leaves, chopped
1–2 tbsp lemon juice

Sweet and tangy miso is a nutritious ingredient that marries beautifully with omega-3-rich salmon fillets. Leaving the fish to marinate overnight ensures it has plenty of flavour and will be moist and tender. Opt for wild salmon, if possible, because it has a higher proportion of omega-3 fats. Serve with stir-fried vegetables.

1 Put the salmon in a shallow ceramic or glass ovenproof dish. Mix together the remaining ingredients, except the coriander and lemon juice, then pour over the fish to coat thoroughly. Cover with cling film and leave to marinate in the fridge overnight.

2 Preheat the oven to 200°C/400°F/Gas 6. Remove the cling film, cover the dish with foil and put into the oven. Cook for 15 minutes. Remove the foil then cook for a further 5–10 minutes until the fish is cooked through. Scatter over the coriander leaves and drizzle with lemon juice to taste before serving. (Store in the fridge for up to 2 days.)

NUTRITIONAL INFORMATION PER SERVING
Protein 32.5g, **Carbohydrates** 7.1g of which sugars 3.6g, **Fat** 17.4g of which saturates 2.9g, **Kcals** 324

HEALTH BENEFITS
Miso provides a good source of protective phytonutrients and antioxidants, including zinc and manganese.

Mixed Seafood Pie

A classic fish pie with a healthy difference: the mixture of seafood is topped with an antioxidant-rich sweet potato mash enriched with tahini. For a dairy-free pie use soya, coconut or oat milk and cream. Serve with a crisp leafy green salad or lightly steamed broccoli and carrots.

1 Preheat the oven to 180°C/350°F/Gas 4. To make the topping, boil the sweet potatoes for 10–15 minutes until tender. Drain and set aside. Meanwhile, heat 1 tablespoon of the olive oil in a large frying pan over medium heat. Add the onion and leek, and gently fry for 5 minutes. Add the fish to the pan and gently fry for 1–2 minutes to seal.

2 Heat the remaining olive oil in a saucepan over medium heat. Stir in the flour and cook for 1 minute. Remove from the heat and gradually beat in the milk and cream. Return to the heat and bring to the boil, whisking constantly. Add the mustard, dill and nutmeg, then season.

3 Stir the fish, vegetables and prawns into the sauce, then spoon into a baking dish. Mash the sweet potato and beat in the cream and tahini, then season. Spoon the mash over the fish. Bake for 20–30 minutes until golden. Serve. (Store in the fridge for up to 2 days or freeze, uncooked, for 1 month.)

SERVES 4
PREPARATION TIME 15 minutes
COOKING TIME 45 minutes

2 tbsp olive oil or coconut oil
1 onion, finely chopped
1 leek, thinly sliced
200g/7oz salmon fillet, skinned and cut into cubes
200g/7oz white fish fillet, such as coley or haddock, skinned and cut into cubes
30g/1oz/¼ cup plain flour
400ml/14fl oz/generous 1½ cups semi-skimmed milk or dairy-free milk
2 tbsp single cream, or oat or soya cream
4 tsp wholegrain mustard
1 handful of dill leaves, chopped
a pinch of freshly grated nutmeg
150g/5½oz peeled cooked prawns
sea salt and freshly ground black pepper

Sweet potato topping
600g/1lb 5oz sweet potatoes, cut into chunks
2 tbsp single cream, or oat or soya cream
1 tbsp tahini

NUTRITIONAL INFORMATION PER SERVING
Protein 34.6g, **Carbohydrates** 37.3g of which sugars 10.5g, **Fat** 18.3g of which saturates 7.6g, **Kcals** 454

HEALTH BENEFITS
Sweet potatoes are rich in antioxidants especially carotenoids and vitamins A and C.

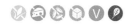

Roasted Tempeh with Piperade Sauce

SERVES 4
PREPARATION TIME 15 minutes
COOKING TIME 30 minutes

2 tbsp olive oil or coconut oil
2 red onions, sliced
6 garlic cloves, chopped
300g/10½oz roasted red peppers from a jar, drained and chopped
4 vine-ripened tomatoes, roughly chopped
1 tbsp sun-dried tomato paste
a pinch of smoked or regular paprika
3 tbsp apple cider vinegar or sherry vinegar
450g/1lb tempeh, cut into 2cm/¾in cubes
olive oil, for drizzling
3 tbsp roughly chopped parsley leaves (optional)
sea salt and freshly ground black pepper

Peppers, garlic, tomatoes and onions form the base of the piperade. If you can find sherry vinegar, its flavour and potent antioxidant and anti-inflammatory qualities will add to the dish. The tempeh readily absorbs the rich flavours of this sauce while it's cooking. Serve with salad.

1 Preheat the oven to 190°C/375°F/Gas 5. Heat a frying pan over medium heat and add 1 tablespoon of the olive oil. Fry the onions for 2 minutes or until just softened. Add the garlic, peppers, tomatoes, tomato paste and paprika, and continue to cook over a gentle heat for 5 minutes or until soft.

2 Put the mixture into a food processor and pulse briefly until coarsely chopped – the mixture should still be chunky. Stir in the vinegar.

3 Heat the remaining oil in the frying pan and add the tempeh. Cook for 10–12 minutes, turning occasionally, until golden. Tip the tempeh into a baking dish and pour over the sauce. Drizzle over a little olive oil and roast for 15 minutes or until the sauce is thick and bubbling. Stir in the parsley, if using, season and serve. (Store in the fridge for up to 2 days.)

NUTRITIONAL INFORMATION PER SERVING
Protein 25.4g, **Carbohydrates** 16.7g of which sugars 9.9g, **Fat** 13.1g of which saturates 4.2g, **Kcals** 291

HEALTH BENEFITS
Tempeh is a highly nutritious fermented food made from soya beans, with a high protein content. It has been a staple in Indonesia for over 2,000 years. Tempeh is rich in essential fatty acids and numerous vitamins, minerals and health-promoting isoflavones.

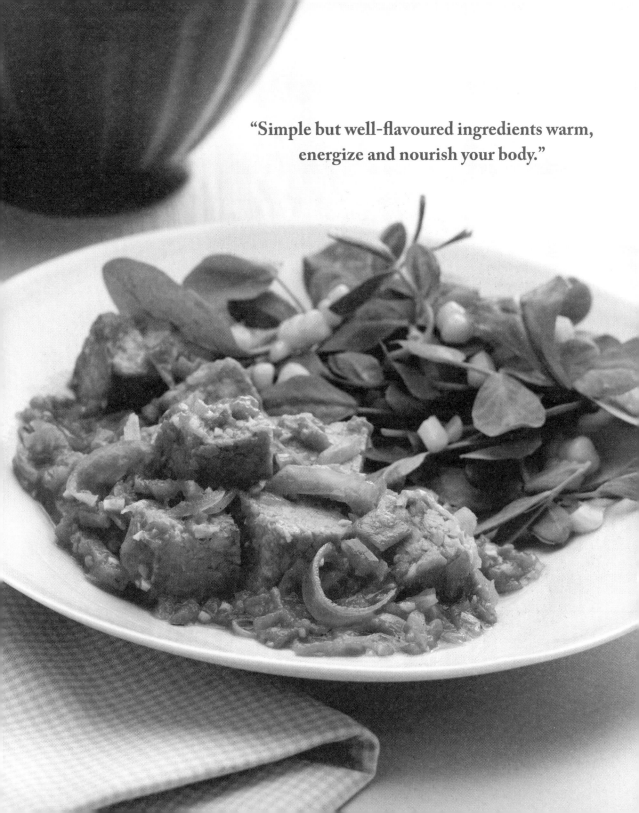

"Simple but well-flavoured ingredients warm, energize and nourish your body."

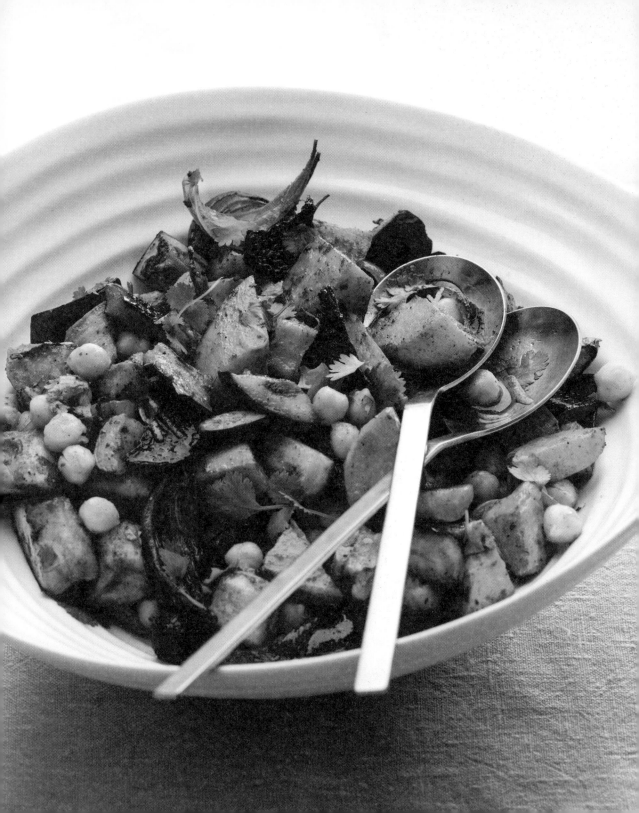

Warm Aubergine, Roots & Chickpea Salad

Cumin and paprika make a tangy, spicy dressing to add to a robust warm salad of roasted vegetables and chickpeas. If you prefer a little extra protein, you can also serve it with some hard-boiled egg, tofu or feta cheese – or, for non-vegetarians, serve with some chicken.

1 Preheat the oven to 200°C/400°F/Gas 6. Put the onion, sweet potato, carrots and beetroots into a baking dish. Mix together the oil, spices, garlic, lemon zest and juice. Pour it over the vegetables and toss to coat.

2 Roast for 15 minutes. Add the aubergines to the baking dish and toss to coat in the oil. Bake for a further 15 minutes or until the vegetables are tender and lightly golden. Remove from the oven. Tip the chickpeas into the baking dish with the coriander.

3 Mix together the dressing ingredients. Drizzle the dressing over the vegetables to serve. (Store in the fridge for up to 2 days.)

SERVES 4
PREPARATION TIME 10 minutes
COOKING TIME 30 minutes

1 red onion, cut into wedges
1 sweet potato, cut into chunks
2 carrots, cut into large chunks
2 small beetroots, cut into wedges
2 tbsp olive oil or melted coconut oil
1 tsp each paprika and ground cumin
1 garlic clove, crushed
zest and juice of ½ lemon
2 aubergines, cut into chunks
400g/14oz/scant 2 cups tinned chickpeas, drained and rinsed
3 tbsp roughly chopped coriander leaves

Spicy dressing
½ tsp ground cumin
a pinch of paprika
2 tsp raw honey or manuka honey
juice of 1 lemon
4 tbsp olive oil or flaxseed oil

NUTRITIONAL INFORMATION PER SERVING
Protein 7.2g, **Carbohydrates** 31.7g of which sugars 15.2g, **Fat** 16.1g of which saturates 5.5g, **Kcals** 298

HEALTH BENEFITS
Aubergines, beetroots and other purple-coloured fruits and vegetables contain anthocyanins, which have been shown to attack cancer cells. Chickpeas, like other beans and pulses, are a good source of phytoestrogens (plant oestrogens) shown to protect against the spread of hormonally driven cancers.

Spaghetti with Lemon & Broccoli

SERVES 4
PREPARATION TIME 10 minutes
COOKING TIME 10 minutes

300g/10½oz wholewheat or spelt
   spaghetti
1kg/2lb 4oz broccoli, cut into small florets
1 tbsp olive oil or coconut oil
2 garlic cloves, crushed
2 red chillies, deseeded and finely
   chopped (optional)
4 spring onions, thinly sliced
zest of 1 lemon
200g/7oz feta cheese, crumbled
juice of ½ lemon
freshly ground black pepper

A simple, fast dish containing broccoli, garlic, chilli and onions – all of which are beneficial for the recovery from cancer. The addition of feta cheese provides protein, but for a dairy-free option, add cooked chicken breast or tinned mixed beans, drained and rinsed.

1 Cook the pasta in boiling water for 7–8 minutes until tender but with a little bite, or according to the packet instructions. Drain.
2 Meanwhile, put the broccoli in a steamer and steam over high heat for 3 minutes or until just tender. Set aside.
3 Heat a frying pan over medium heat and add the olive oil. Gently fry the garlic, chillies, if using, onions and lemon zest for 2–3 minutes until just softened. Add the broccoli and heat through. Tip the broccoli mixture into the pasta with the feta cheese and lemon juice and toss well. Season with black pepper, then serve. (Store in the fridge for up to 1 day.)

NUTRITIONAL INFORMATION PER SERVING
Protein 29.1g, **Carbohydrates** 51.6g of which sugars 7.3g, **Fat** 16.5g of which saturates 9.6g, **Kcals** 474

HEALTH BENEFITS
Both wholewheat and spelt spaghetti have a lower glycaemic index than white pasta, meaning that the effect on blood sugar levels is reduced, and they also provide a useful source of dietary fibre.

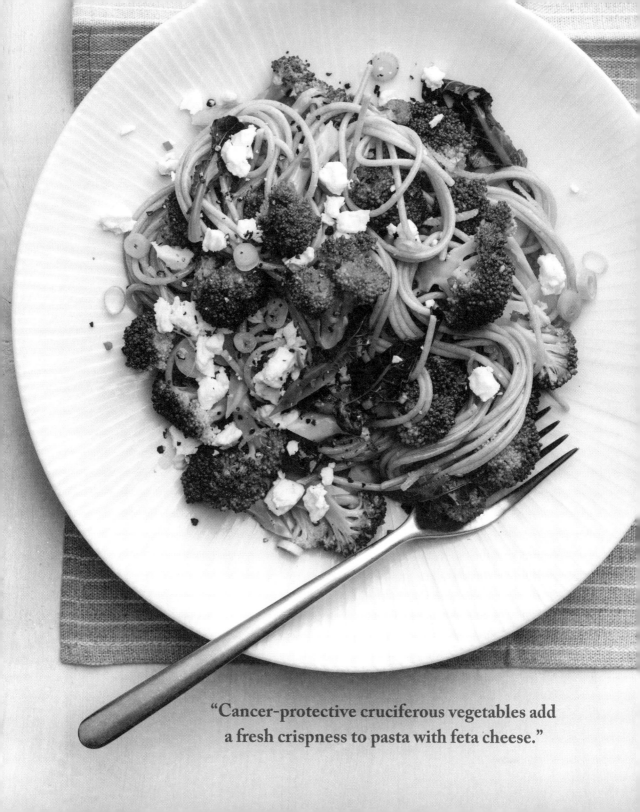

"Cancer-protective cruciferous vegetables add a fresh crispness to pasta with feta cheese."

Hemp Seed & Nut Burgers

SERVES 4

PREPARATION TIME 10 minutes,
  plus 30 minutes chilling

COOKING TIME 40 minutes

1 tbsp olive oil or coconut oil
1 red onion, finely chopped
1 carrot, grated
90g/3¼oz mushrooms, finely chopped
1 garlic clove, crushed
115g/4oz/heaped ½ cup tinned cannellini
  beans, drained and rinsed
50g/1¾oz/scant ½ cup walnut pieces
50g/1¾oz/⅓ cup cashew nuts
2 tbsp shelled hemp seeds
60g/2¼oz/¾ cup fresh wholemeal
  breadcrumbs, or gluten-free
  breadcrumbs or oats
1 tbsp tamari
2 tsp raw honey
1 egg yolk
sea salt and freshly ground black pepper

Home-made vegetarian burgers taste wholesome and satisfying. Full of fibre, protein and healthy fats, these hemp seed and nut burgers make a popular family meal, and because they can be frozen, they are useful to make ahead for those days when a quickly cooked meal is all you fancy. Serve with a salad and some salsa or Celeriac, Apple & Fennel Remoulade (page 88).

1 Heat the olive oil in a large frying pan over medium heat and add the onion, carrot, mushrooms and garlic. Gently fry for 10 minutes or until the vegetables are soft and the liquid has evaporated. Add the beans to the pan and cook for 1 minute. Leave the mixture to cool slightly.

2 Put the nuts in a food processor and pulse until coarsely chopped. Add the bean mixture and the remaining ingredients, and pulse to combine. Chill for 30 minutes. Preheat the oven to 190°C/375°F/Gas 5 and line a baking tray with baking parchment.

3 Shape the mixture into 8 burgers. Put on to the baking tray and bake for 20–30 minutes until crisp and golden. Serve. (Store in the fridge for up to 3 days or freeze, uncooked, for up to 3 months.)

NUTRITIONAL INFORMATION PER SERVING
Protein 5.9g, **Carbohydrates** 11.4g of which sugars 3.3g, **Fat** 11.1g of which saturates 1.6g, **Kcals** 169

HEALTH BENEFITS
Using hemp seeds and nuts in these vegetarian burgers increases their protein content and provides essential omega-3 and -6 fats. Walnuts are also rich in antioxidant phenols and vitamin E. They are a valuable anti-cancer food and their consumption has been shown to reduce the risk of certain cancers, including prostate and breast cancer.

Persian Quinoa Omega Bowl

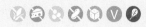

This versatile Middle Eastern-inspired salad is packed with colourful vegetables, grains and pulses, pomegranate seeds and berries, plus omega-rich seeds and oils. Add a poached egg or some feta cheese if you would like to have more protein. Leftovers make a good packed lunch.

1 Preheat the oven to 180°C/350°F/Gas 4. Put the aubergine, pepper and squash into a baking dish and toss with the 3 tablespoons olive oil and the cumin. Season and cook in the oven for 30 minutes or until tender.

2 Meanwhile, put the quinoa into a saucepan with 375ml/ 13fl oz/1½ cups water and the saffron, if using. Bring to the boil, cover and reduce the heat to a very low simmer. Cook for 15 minutes, then turn off the heat and keep covered for a further 5 minutes.

3 Put the green beans in a steamer and steam over high heat for 2 minutes. Drain and refresh under cold water. Tip the quinoa into a large bowl and add the cooked vegetables, lentils, seeds, berries and tomatoes.

4 Mix together the olive oil, the lemon zest and juice, and mint. Pour it over the salad and toss to coat before serving. (Store in the fridge for up to 3 days.)

SERVES 6

PREPARATION TIME 15 minutes

COOKING TIME 30 minutes

1 small aubergine, cut into 2cm/¾in chunks

1 red pepper, deseeded and cut into chunks

200g/7oz butternut squash, diced

3 tbsp olive oil

1 tsp cumin seeds

150g/5½oz/scant 1 cup quinoa

½ tsp saffron threads (optional)

100g/3½oz green beans, cut in half

400g/14oz/2 cups tinned Puy lentils, drained and rinsed

6 tbsp mixed seeds, such as sunflower, pumpkin and shelled hemp seeds

3 tbsp pomegranate seeds

3 tbsp dried unsweetened berries

8 cherry tomatoes, cut in half

4 tbsp olive oil or flaxseed oil

zest and juice of 1 lemon

3 tbsp chopped mint leaves

sea salt and freshly ground black pepper

NUTRITIONAL INFORMATION PER SERVING

Protein 14.6g, **Carbohydrates** 33.5g of which sugars 13g, **Fat** 27.1g of which saturates 3g, **Kcals** 442

HEALTH BENEFITS

Quinoa is a nutritious gluten-free grain-like seed that is high in protein, containing all nine essential amino acids. It contains magnesium for energy production and is a source of manganese, which helps to protect cells from oxidative damage.

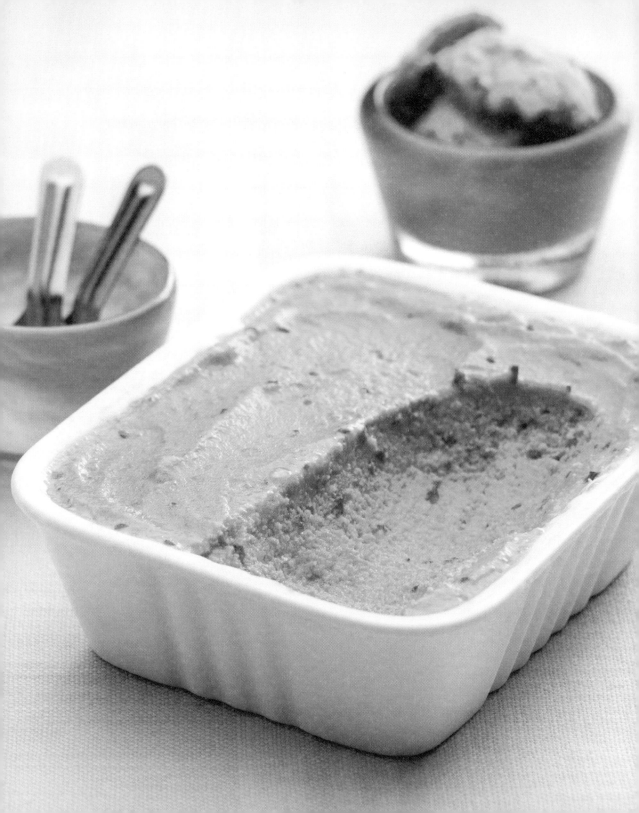

Desserts & Baked Treats

Cancer treatments can often increase the cravings for something sweet, especially for patients who experience a bitter or metallic taste in their mouths. In this chapter you will find a range of low-sugar recipes for desserts as well as baked treats — perfect for travelling and packed lunches. None contain refined sugar and all are carefully balanced to help stabilize blood sugar. Rather than providing empty calories, these dishes are rich with nutritious ingredients and are designed to support your energy levels. There is a whole range of tempting desserts, including Apple, Walnut & Pistachio Crumble, and Gooey Chocolate & Raspberry Pudding. Among the cakes and bakes are Matcha Tea & Banana Cake or, for a savoury option, Savoury Onion Kale Crisps and Spiced Flatbreads.

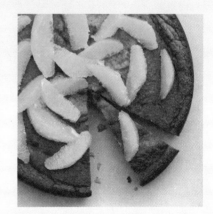

Opposite: Super-Berry Yogurt Sorbet (page 126)
Above: Almond Citrus Cake (page 124)

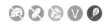

Gooey Chocolate & Raspberry Pudding

SERVES 4
PREPARATION TIME 10 minutes
COOKING TIME 40 minutes

oil, for greasing
125g/4½oz/heaped ¾ cup wholemeal
    plain flour or gluten-free flour mix
2 tsp baking powder
1 tbsp cocoa powder
1 tsp vanilla extract
125g/4½oz/scant ½ cup sugar-free apple
    purée
125ml/4fl oz/½ cup soya milk
1 tbsp xylitol
150g/5½oz/scant 1¼ cups raspberries,
    plus extra to serve (optional)

Chocolate sauce
2 tbsp xylitol
1 heaped tbsp cocoa powder

Beneath a light chocolate sponge studded with fresh raspberries lies an intense chocolate sauce. Perhaps surprisingly, this is a healthy dish, because it uses puréed apple and xylitol to give it a touch of sweetness.

1 Preheat the oven to 180°C/350°F/Gas 4 and lightly grease a 20cm/8in round baking dish. Sift the flour, baking powder and cocoa powder into a bowl, then tip in the bran.

2 Mix together the vanilla, apple purée, milk and xylitol, and beat into the flour mixture. Stir in the raspberries, then spoon into the baking dish.

3 Combine the sauce ingredients with 400ml/14fl oz/ generous 1½ cups boiling water, and pour gently over the batter. Do not stir the liquid in – it will seep in as it cooks.

4 Carefully put the dish in the oven and bake for 35–40 minutes until the pudding is firm on top but with a gooey chocolate sauce underneath. Serve with extra raspberries, if you like. (Store leftovers in the fridge for up to 2 days.)

NUTRITIONAL INFORMATION PER SERVING
Protein 5.4g, **Carbohydrates** 38.7g of which sugars 14.8g, **Fat** 2.2g of which of saturates 0.8g, **Kcals** 181

HEALTH BENEFITS
Polyphenols, in the cocoa powder, are known for their antioxidant properties. For a stronger antioxidant boost you can use high-antioxidant cocoa powder, which is readily available. It has a slightly stronger, bitter taste, so use a little less in the recipe and increase the amount of xylitol slightly.

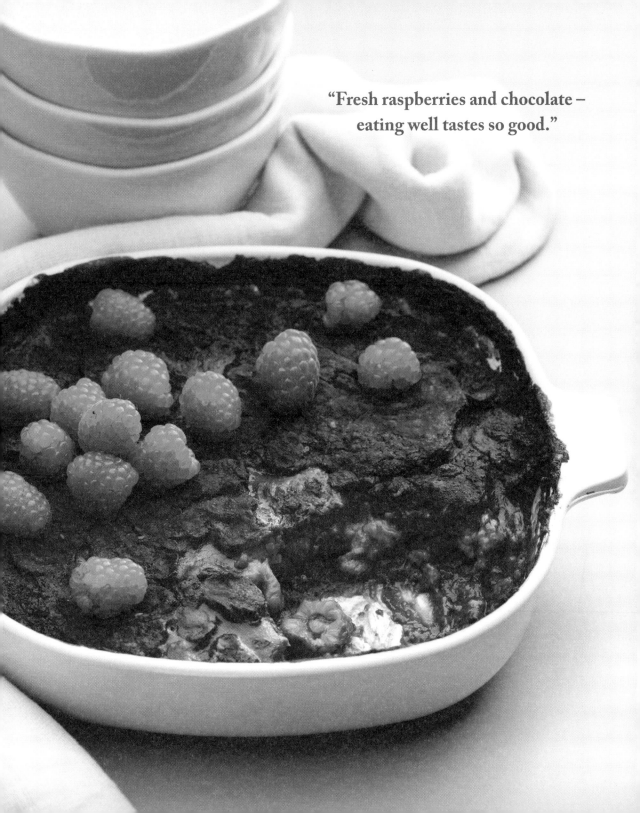

"Fresh raspberries and chocolate –
eating well tastes so good."

Apple, Walnut & Pistachio Crumble

SERVES 8
PREPARATION TIME 15 minutes
COOKING TIME 30 minutes

2 tbsp olive oil or coconut oil, plus extra
    for greasing
1.3kg/3lb cooking apples, such as
    Bramley, peeled and cut into chunks
1 tsp cinnamon
3 tbsp xylitol
1 tbsp apple concentrate or raw honey

Crumble topping
75g/2½oz/heaped ¾ cup unsweetened
    desiccated coconut
115g/4oz/¾ cup pistachio nuts
115g/4oz/scant 1 cup walnut pieces
a pinch of sea salt
60g/2¼oz/⅔ cup porridge oats or
    buckwheat flakes
60g/2¼oz/⅓ cup pitted dried dates

A healthy version of the traditional crumble with a topping of ground nuts and oats sweetened with dates. You don't have to bake it – you can simply sprinkle the crumble mixture over the cooked apples and serve, if you prefer. Natural yogurt goes very well with it.

1   Preheat the oven to 200°C/400°F/Gas 6 and grease a baking dish. Heat a saucepan over medium heat and add the olive oil, apples, cinnamon, xylitol and apple concentrate, then cook for 5–8 minutes until the apples are soft. Add a splash of water, if necessary, to prevent it drying out. Transfer the apples to the dish.
2   To make the crumble, put the coconut, nuts and salt into a food processor and process to form crumbs. Pulse in the oats and dates to form coarse crumbs. Sprinkle the topping over the apples, then bake for 15–20 minutes until golden and bubbling. Serve hot or warm. (Leftovers can be stored in the fridge for up to 2 days.)

NUTRITIONAL INFORMATION PER SERVING
Protein 6.8g, **Carbohydrates** 32.1g of which sugars 27.3g, **Fat** 24.4g of which saturates 7.2g, **Kcals** 368

HEALTH BENEFITS
Apples are rich in polyphenols – antioxidants shown to help balance blood sugar levels and reduce glucose spikes. They also provide soluble fibre, including pectin, which has been shown to help with the excretion of fat and cholesterol from the body.

Baked Lemon Cheesecake

A creamy, dairy-free cheesecake that is low in sugar but high in protein and isoflavones. A little xylitol and some dates provide sweetness, and the cheesecake is served with an antioxidant-rich berry sauce. Behind its indulgent appearance and taste is a healthy dessert that's perfect for entertaining too.

1 Preheat the oven to 180°C/350°F/Gas 4 and lightly grease a 20cm/8in springform cake tin. Put the oatcakes and coconut into a food processor and pulse to form fine crumbs. Add the butter, dates, lemon zest and juice. Process to form a sticky dough. Spoon into the prepared tin and press into the base.

2 Put the filling ingredients into the food processor and process until smooth. Pour over the crumb base, then bake for 35–40 minutes until firm. Turn off the oven and leave to cool in the oven for 30 minutes.

3 Meanwhile, to make the sauce, mix the cornflour with 2 tablespoons water. Put the berries into a saucepan with the cornflour mixture and simmer for 1–2 minutes, stirring, to thicken. Leave to cool. Serve the cheesecake with the sauce. (Store leftovers in the fridge for up to 4 days.)

SERVES 8

PREPARATION TIME 15 minutes

COOKING TIME 45 minutes, plus cooling

60g/2¼oz/¼ cup butter, melted, or melted coconut oil, plus extra for greasing

150g/5½oz rough oatcakes or gluten-free oatcakes

90g/3¼oz/1 cup unsweetened desiccated coconut

60g/2¼oz/⅓ cup pitted dried dates

zest and juice of 1 lemon

Tofu filling

500g/1lb 2oz silken tofu or firm tofu

zest of 4 lemons and juice of 1

60g/2¼oz/⅓ cup xylitol

3 egg yolks

30g/1oz/¼ cup cornflour

Berry sauce

1 tbsp cornflour

250g/9oz/2 cups fresh or frozen mixed berries

NUTRITIONAL INFORMATION PER SERVING

Protein 9.4g, **Carbohydrates** 33.1g of which sugars 15.8g, **Fat** 22.1g of which saturates 14.4g, **Kcals** 359

HEALTH BENEFITS

The tofu and eggs are protein rich and low in sugar. Berries are a good source of phytonutrients, including cancer-protective chemicals such as ellagic acid (richest in strawberries and raspberries) and anthocyanosides (richest in blueberries).

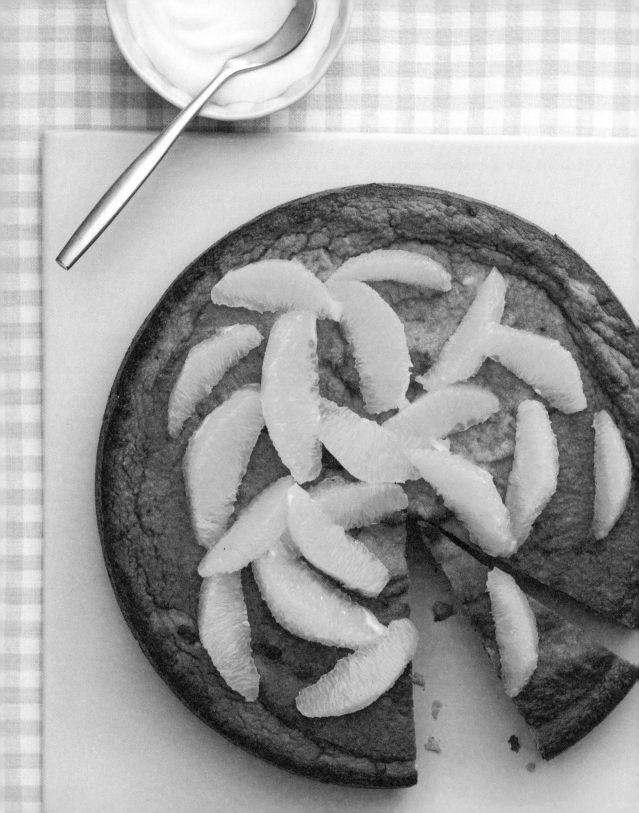

Almond Citrus Cake

The oranges in this moist dessert cake give it a vibrant tang. It can be served warm or cold accompanied with soya or natural yogurt and some orange segments or other fresh fruit. Using olive oil, rich in omega-9, is an easy way to cram healthy anti-inflammatory fats into your diet, and using almonds instead of flour keeps this cake gluten-free and high in protein.

1 Boil the oranges whole for 1½ hours or until soft. Preheat the oven to 180°C/350°F/Gas 4 and grease a 23cm/9in cake tin.
2 Put the whole oranges into a blender or food processor and process until smooth. Add the lemon zest, eggs, xylitol, oil, almonds, salt and bicarbonate of soda, then pulse until thoroughly mixed. Pour the batter into the prepared cake tin.
3 Bake for 45–50 minutes until a skewer inserted into the centre comes out clean. Leave to cool in the tin before turning out. Serve with fresh fruit, if you like. (Store, wrapped, in the fridge for up to 3 days or freeze for up to 3 months.)

SERVES 12
PREPARATION TIME 10 minutes
COOKING TIME 2 hours 20 minutes, plus cooling

2 oranges, washed
3 tbsp olive oil, plus extra for greasing
zest of 1 lemon
4 eggs
60g/2¼oz/⅓ cup xylitol
250g/9oz/2½ cups ground almonds
½ tsp sea salt
1 tsp bicarbonate of soda
fresh fruit, to serve (optional)

NUTRITIONAL INFORMATION PER SERVING
Protein 6.7g, **Carbohydrates** 7.9g of which sugars 7.2g, **Fat** 15.8g of which saturates 1.8g, **Kcals** 193

HEALTH BENEFITS
Using the oranges whole, including the peel, retains the citrus flavanones, which tend to be concentrated around the pith and peel. These phytonutrients have been shown to be particularly powerful against many types of cancers.

Green Tea Ice Cream

SERVES 6

PREPARATION TIME 10 minutes,
  plus 2 hours freezing

115g/4oz/¾ cup cashew nuts

30g/1oz/¼ cup plain or vanilla protein
  powder (such as whey or rice) (optional)

200ml/7fl oz/scant 1 cup coconut water
  or water

1 tbsp raw or manuka honey (optional)

3 mint leaves

1 tsp matcha green tea powder

4 bananas, sliced and frozen

1 Put all the ingredients, except the bananas, into a blender or food processor. Process until smooth. Add the bananas and process. Serve at once or freeze. (Store in the freezer for up to 3 months; allow to soften slightly before serving.)

NUTRITIONAL INFORMATION PER SERVING
Protein 6.8g, **Carbohydrates** 23.7g of which sugars 17.9g,
Fat 10.1g of which saturates 2g, **Kcals** 214

HEALTH BENEFITS
Matcha is exceptionally high in antioxidants and contains a potent class of antioxidant known as catechins. Green tea is also rich in L-theanine, an amino acid that promotes a state of relaxation and well-being by creating alpha waves in the brain.

Super-Berry Yogurt Sorbet ▶

SERVES 4

PREPARATION TIME: 5 minutes,
  plus 3 hours freezing

200g/7oz/generous ¾ cup natural yogurt,
  soya yogurt or coconut yogurt

2 tsp acai berry powder (optional)

125g/4½oz/heaped ¾ cup strawberries

125g/4½oz/1 cup raspberries

225g/8oz/heaped 1 cup fresh or frozen
  cherries, pitted

1 Put all the ingredients into a blender or food processor and process until smooth. Pour into a shallow freezerproof container and freeze for 2–3 hours until firm. Remove from the freezer 30 minutes before serving to allow it to soften slightly. (Store in the freezer for up to 3 months.)

NUTRITIONAL INFORMATION PER SERVING
Protein 4g, **Carbohydrates** 12.2g of which sugars 11.5g,
Fat 5.3g of which saturates 3.4g, **Kcals** 110

HEALTH BENEFITS
The probiotic natural yogurt supports your immune system and digestive health. The optional acai berry powder provides additional antioxidant benefits.

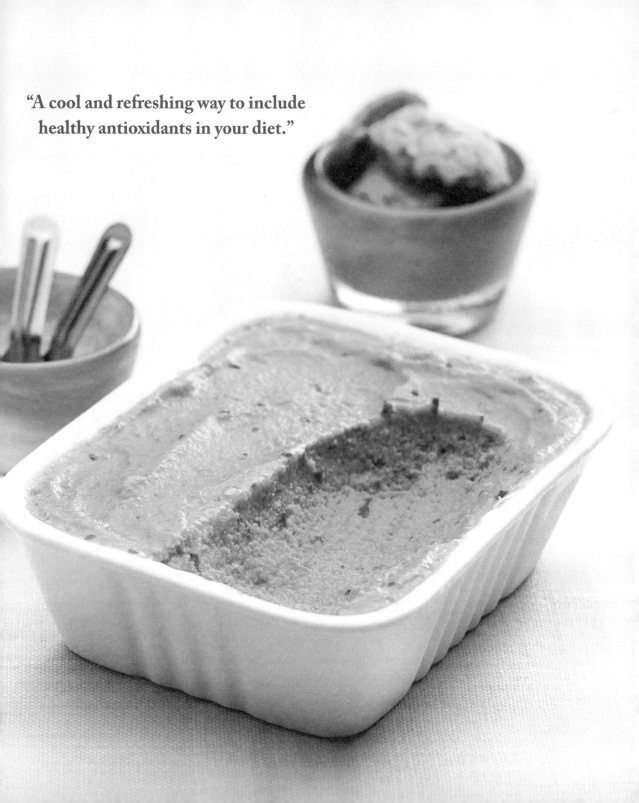

"A cool and refreshing way to include healthy antioxidants in your diet."

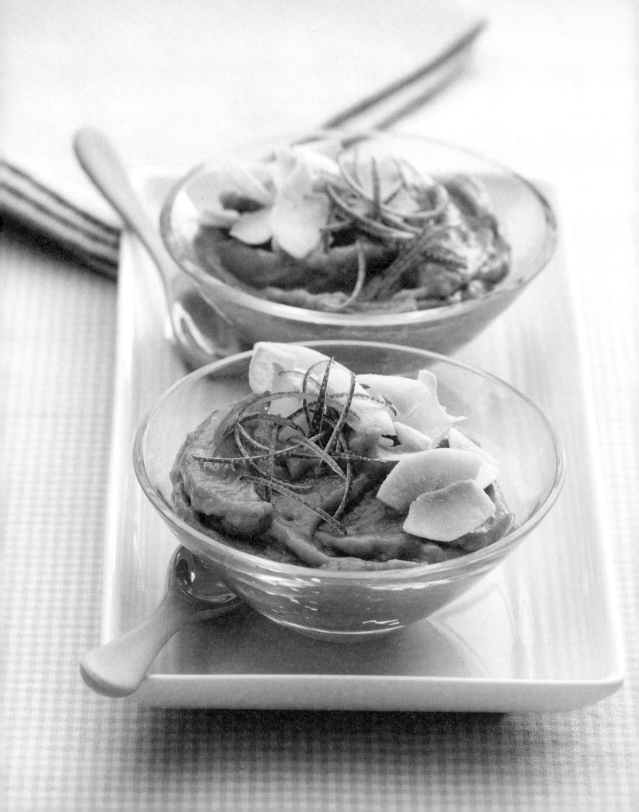

Avocado Lime Mousse

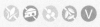

Tangy, zesty and refreshing, this simple dessert combines lime juice with creamy avocado and sweet dates to create a sensational but healthy mousse. Qualities include good fats, vitamins E and C, beta-carotenes and phytonutrients. The mousse can be prepared in advance and chilled until needed.

SERVES 4

PREPARATION TIME 5 minutes, plus 1–2 hours chilling

2 whole limes
juice of 2 limes
2 ripe avocados, pitted and peeled
125g/4½oz/heaped ⅔ cup pitted dried dates
1 tbsp raw honey or manuka honey (optional)
2 tbsp unsweetened coconut flakes, to serve

1 With a sharp knife, remove the zest in strips from the whole limes and remove any pips. Reserve the zest. Put the limes and the remaining ingredients into a blender or food processor and process until smooth and creamy.

2 Spoon into 4 individual dishes and chill for 1–2 hours before serving. Cut the zest into fine strips, and use to decorate the mousses, then top with a sprinkling of coconut flakes before serving. (Store in the fridge for up to 1 day.)

NUTRITIONAL INFORMATION PER SERVING
Protein 2.5g, **Carbohydrates** 21.4g of which sugars 21.2g, **Fat** 13g of which saturates 4.8g, **Kcals** 213

HEALTH BENEFITS
Avocados contain B vitamins, including folate and B6. The optional manuka honey is well known for its anti-bacterial and anti-fungal properties and is useful for soothing sore throats, ulcers and wounds as well as supporting energy levels and aiding digestion. The active ingredient found in manuka but not present in other honeys is known as UMF (unique manuka factor).

Matcha Tea & Banana Cake

MAKES 1 cake, 10 slices

PREPARATION TIME 15 minutes

COOKING TIME 45 minutes, plus cooling

125g/4½oz/½ cup unsalted butter, melted, or melted coconut oil, plus extra for greasing

150g/5½oz/1 cup wholemeal self-raising flour, or gluten-free flour mix plus ½ tsp xanthan gum

2 tsp matcha green tea powder or 1 tbsp ground green tea leaves

2 tsp baking powder

1 tsp cinnamon

3 tbsp ground flaxseed

4 tbsp unsweetened desiccated coconut

90g/3¼oz/½ cup ready-to-eat dried apricots, chopped

3 bananas, mashed

2 eggs

50g/1¾oz/scant ⅓ cup xylitol

An antioxidant-packed version of an all-time favourite, containing matcha – powdered green tea. This recipe is much lower in sugar than traditional teacakes, using fresh and dried fruit for sweetness.

1 Preheat the oven to 180°C/350°F/Gas 4, then grease and base-line a 450g/1lb loaf tin with baking parchment. Sift the flour, matcha, baking powder and cinnamon into a bowl and tip in any bran remaining in the sieve. Stir in the flaxseed, 2 tablespoons of the coconut and the chopped apricots.

2 Pour the melted butter into a blender or food processor, add the bananas, eggs and xylitol, and process until smooth. Add to the flour mixture and stir thoroughly. Spoon the mixture into the loaf tin and sprinkle over the remaining coconut.

3 Bake for 40–45 minutes until firm and golden – a skewer inserted into the centre will come out clean. If the top begins to brown too much, cover with foil. Leave to cool in the tin for 10 minutes, then turn out on to a wire rack to cool completely before serving. (Store, wrapped, in the fridge for up to 3 days or freeze for 1 month.)

NUTRITIONAL INFORMATION PER SLICE
Protein 5.8g, **Carbohydrates** 24.2g of which sugars 13.9g, **Fat** 15.1g of which saturates 8.4g, **Kcals** 247

HEALTH BENEFITS
Eating matcha – the whole leaf of green tea – gives you the benefit of its plentiful antioxidants. Using wholemeal flour and ground flaxseed adds nutrients including lignans, omega-3 fats and soluble fibre. The B vitamins, magnesium and selenium boost energy levels.

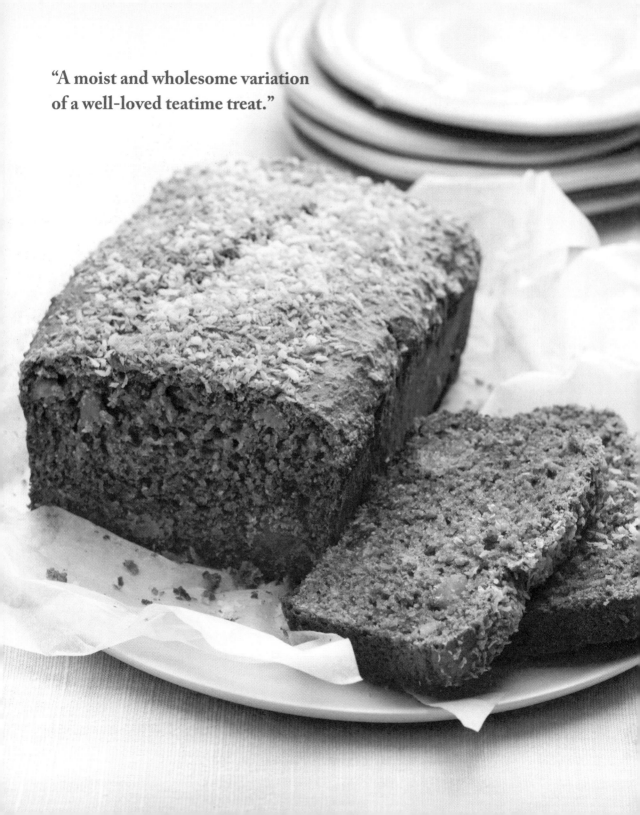

"A moist and wholesome variation of a well-loved teatime treat."

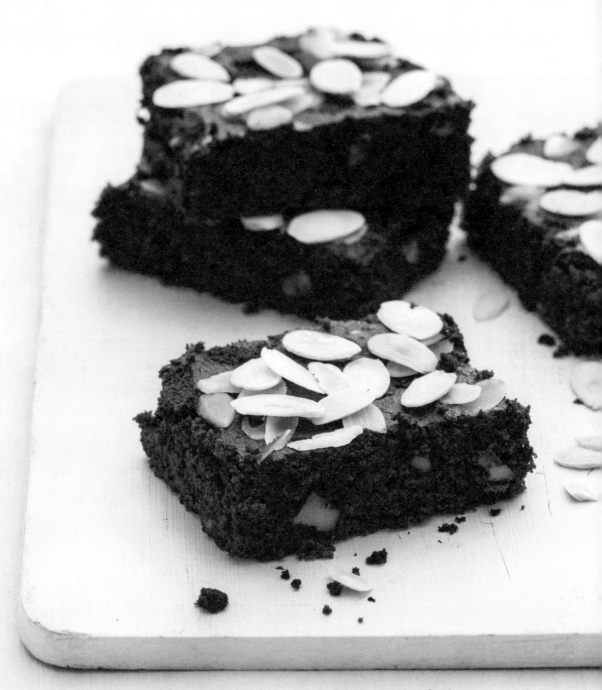

"The nourishing answer when you're feeling tired and prefer to eat something sweet."

Chocolate Beetroot Traybake

MAKES 10

PREPARATION TIME 10 minutes

COOKING TIME 30 minutes,
plus cooling

60g/2¼oz/¼ cup butter or coconut oil,
plus extra for greasing

250g/9oz dairy-free dark chocolate

3 tbsp xylitol

4 eggs

1 large cooked beetroot (about
150g/5½oz), roughly chopped

100g/3½oz/1 cup ground almonds

a pinch of sea salt

½ tsp cinnamon

½ tsp bicarbonate of soda

60g/2¼oz/scant ½ cup walnut pieces,
chopped

30g/1oz/⅓ cup flaked almonds

This traybake is similar to a chocolate brownie but much healthier and the perfect pick-me-up to restore flagging energy levels. Beetroot is added to chocolate cakes because of the soft and moist crumb it produces, and here it is combined with nuts to add flavour and texture.

1 Preheat the oven to 180°C/350°F/Gas 4, then grease a shallow 20 × 30cm/8 × 12in traybake tin and line with baking parchment. Put the chocolate, xylitol and butter into a saucepan and heat gently to melt the chocolate. Put the eggs and beetroot into a blender or food processor and process until smooth.

2 Tip the ground almonds into a large bowl. Add the melted chocolate mixture, the beetroot mixture and the remaining ingredients except the flaked almonds. Mix well.

3 Pour the batter into the tin, then scatter over the flaked almonds. Bake for 20–25 minutes until firm and the almonds are golden. Leave to cool in the tin on a wire rack, then cut into bars to serve. (Store in an airtight container in the fridge for up to 4 days or freeze for 1 month.)

NUTRITIONAL INFORMATION PER BAR

Protein 7.7g, **Carbohydrates** 21.1g of which sugars 20.6g, **Fat** 26.6g of which saturates 11g, **Kcals** 349

HEALTH BENEFITS

The almonds and walnuts increase the protein content, which helps to balance blood sugar. They also supply healthy fats, vitamins and minerals, including manganese, vitamin E, calcium and magnesium. Beetroots are rich in cancer-protective nutrients including antioxidants such as betalains, which have been shown to lessen tumour cell growth.

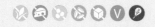

Savoury Onion Kale Crisps

SERVES 8
PREPARATION TIME 10 minutes
COOKING TIME 20 minutes,
  plus cooling

oil, for greasing
200g/7oz curly kale, stems removed, cut
  into large pieces
60g/2¼oz/heaped ⅓ cup cashew nuts
2 tbsp nutritional yeast flakes or
  1 tsp garlic powder
1 small onion, roughly chopped
½ tsp turmeric
2 tbsp apple cider vinegar
1 tsp sea salt

These healthy kale crisps have a taste of cheese but are in fact dairy-free – the flavour comes from using nutritional yeast flakes. Adding turmeric to the mix creates a golden glaze to the kale and adds cancer-protective curcumin.

1 Preheat the oven to 180°C/350°F/Gas 4 and lightly grease 2 baking sheets. Put the kale in a large bowl. Put the remaining ingredients into a blender or food processor and process to create a thick sauce. You may need to add 1–2 tablespoons water to thin the mixture.

2 Pour the mixture over the kale and use your hands to massage the sauce into the kale leaves so that they are thoroughly coated. Arrange the kale, spaced apart, on the baking sheets.

3 Bake for 15–20 minutes, turning twice during cooking to ensure they become crisp. Remove from the oven and leave to cool before serving. (Store in an airtight container for up to 3 days.)

NUTRITIONAL INFORMATION PER SERVING
Protein 3.6g, **Carbohydrates** 3.1g of which sugars 1.1g, **Fat** 4.2g of which saturates 0.8g, **Kcals** 64

HEALTH BENEFITS
The nutritional yeast flakes are a good source of B vitamins. Kale contains cancer-protective nutrients, particularly glucosinolates, which are converted into isothiocyanates in the body, and have been shown to protect against bladder, breast, colon, ovary and prostate cancers. Kale also contains flavonoids, including kaempferol and quercetin, which possess important antioxidant and anti-inflammatory benefits helping lower inflammation and oxidative stress.

Spiced Flatbreads

Middle Eastern baked flatbreads make a perfect accompaniment to curries, soups and stews. Lightly spiced with cumin, these have the added health benefits of including turmeric too.

MAKES 4

SERVES 8

PREPARATION TIME 25 minutes, plus 1¼ hours rising

COOKING TIME 10 minutes, plus cooling

1 tbsp cumin seeds

15g/½oz dried yeast

1 tbsp raw honey

250g/9oz/2 cups strong white bread flour

250g/9oz/1⅔ cups strong wholemeal bread flour

2 tsp turmeric

1 tsp salt

2 tbsp olive oil, plus extra for greasing

1 tbsp sesame seeds

1 Toast the cumin seeds in a dry frying pan over medium heat until fragrant. Grind using a mortar and pestle. Put the yeast and honey in a jug with 150ml/5fl oz/scant ⅔ cup lukewarm water and stir to dissolve. Leave for 10 minutes or until frothy.

2 Sift the flours, turmeric, salt and cumin into a large bowl. Gradually pour in the yeast mixture. Add 150ml/5fl oz/scant ⅔ cup lukewarm water and the olive oil, and mix to form a soft dough. Knead for 5 minutes or until smooth.

3 Put the dough in a greased bowl and cover with cling film. Leave for 1 hour or until doubled in size. Preheat the oven to 220°C/425°F/Gas 7.

4 Divide the dough into 4. Roll into oval shapes 2cm/¾in thick. Brush with a little water and sprinkle with sesame seeds. Bake direct on the oven shelf for 7–10 minutes until puffed up. Transfer to a wire rack to cool slightly, and serve warm, or leave to cool completely. (Store, wrapped, in the fridge for up to 3 days or freeze for 1 month.)

NUTRITIONAL INFORMATION PER SERVING (½ FLATBREAD)
Protein 16.1g, **Carbohydrates** 86.7g of which sugars 6.5g, **Fat** 9.2g of which saturates 1.4g, **Kcals** 493

HEALTH BENEFITS
The combination of wholemeal and plain flours increases the nutritional profile and soluble fibre of the flatbreads. Turmeric contains curcumin, which possesses anti-inflammatory properties and is also cancer-protective.

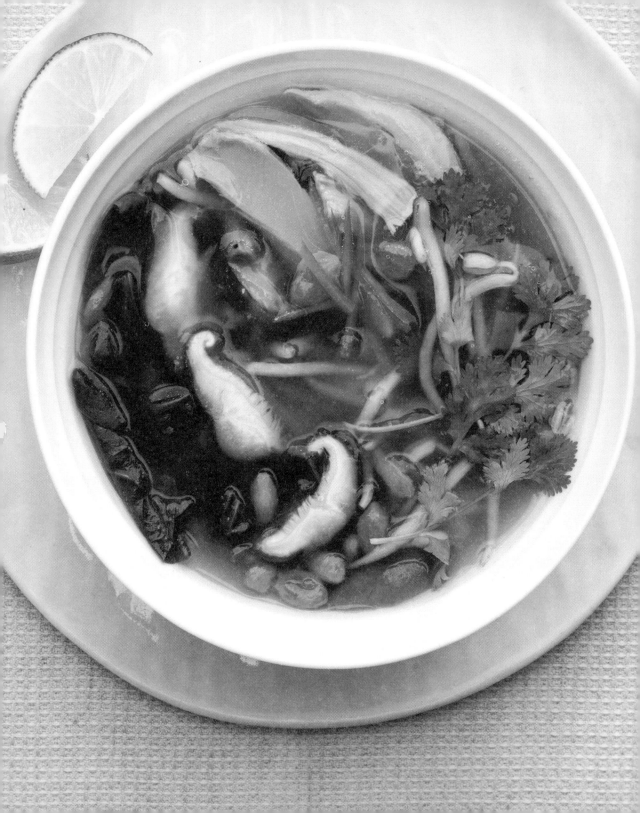

Supporting Your Body through Treatment

Whether in combination with conventional cancer treatment or alone, good nutrition can help to enhance your healing. A healthier diet may also alleviate some of the common side effects of the disease and/or the treatment. Incorporating certain key foods and herbs in your meals can assist you through your treatment and help your recovery. In this chapter you will find recipes designed to counter the symptoms of nausea, a loss of appetite, weight loss, low immune function, fatigue and digestive problems. Boost your energy with our Wheatgrass Energizer, snack on our Ginger, Almond & Chocolate Cookies to help manage nausea, or support your immune health with our delicious Noodle, Shallot & Shiitake Salad.

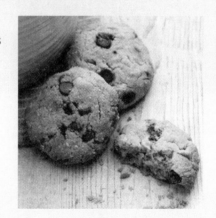

Opposite: Chicken Ginger Miso Soup (page 146)
Above: Ginger, Almond & Chocolate Cookies (page 140)

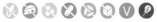

Ginger Vegetable Juice ▶

SERVES 2, 250ml/9fl oz/1 cup each
PREPARATION TIME 5 minutes

2 carrots
½ cucumber
2 celery sticks
1 lemon, peeled
3 apples
2cm/¾in piece of fresh root ginger
ice cubes, to serve (optional)

1 Put all the ingredients through an electric juicer. Mix well and serve over ice, if you like. Drink immediately.

NUTRITIONAL INFORMATION PER SERVING
Protein 2g, **Carbohydrates** 19g of which sugars 18.9g,
Fat 0.6g of which saturates 0.1g, **Kcals** 91

HEALTH BENEFITS
Cucumber is an excellent hydrator and contains lignans, which may be effective against certain types of cancers. The minerals potassium and sodium are present in celery and are important for regulating fluid balance.

    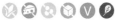

Gazpacho Smoothie

SERVES 1, 250ml/9fl oz/1 cup
PREPARATION TIME 5 minutes

3 vine-ripened tomatoes
½ cucumber
1 tbsp chopped coriander leaves
½ garlic clove, chopped
1 dash of cayenne pepper, or to taste
¼ tsp ground cumin
1 tsp flaxseed oil
1 tbsp lime juice
1 ripe pear, peeled and chopped
1 tbsp seeds or nuts, to serve

1 Put all the ingredients into a blender or food processor and process until smooth. Add a little water to thin if needed. Drink immediately or store in the fridge for up to 1 day. Serve with 1 tablespoon seeds or nuts.

NUTRITIONAL INFORMATION PER SERVING
Protein 6.4g, **Carbohydrates** 23.6g of which sugars 21.8g,
Fat 12.4g of which saturates 1.7g, **Kcals** 237

HEALTH BENEFITS
Keeping yourself hydrated and nourished is important in controlling feelings of nausea. This smoothie is rich in electrolytes – sodium and potassium – which can help to settle the stomach and re-energize you.

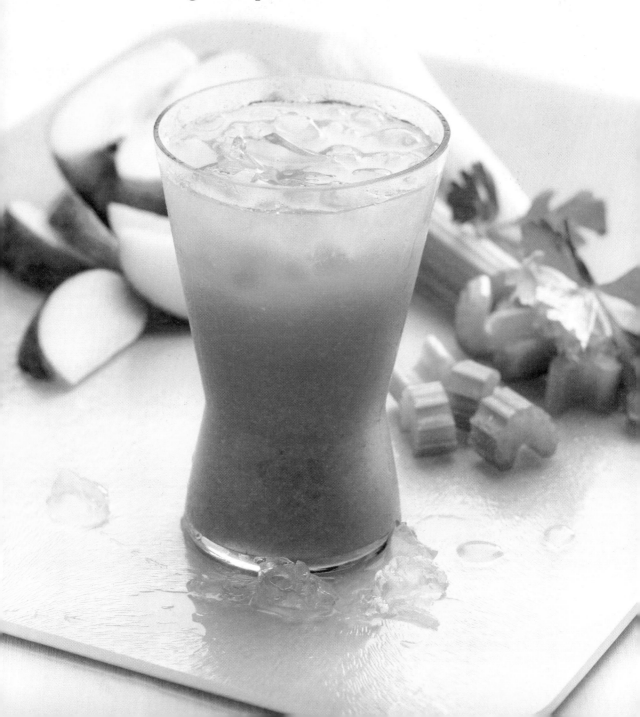

"Ginger is a remarkable natural aid to relieve digestive upsets and nausea."

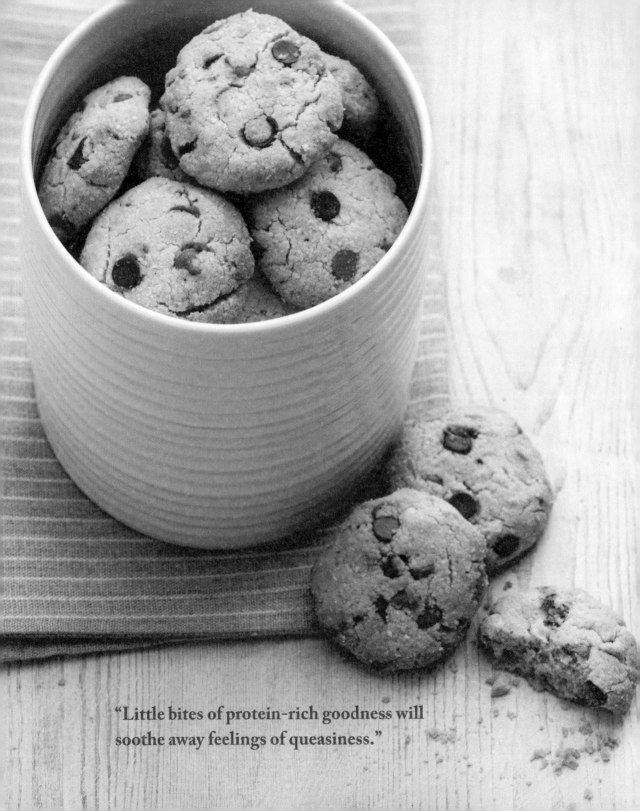

"Little bites of protein-rich goodness will soothe away feelings of queasiness."

Ginger, Almond & Chocolate Cookies

These soft cookies are ideal to snack on when you feel nauseous or your appetite is low. The perfect combination of ginger and chocolate makes them particularly tempting.

1 Preheat the oven to 190°C/375°F/Gas 5 and line a baking sheet with baking parchment. Put the almonds in a bowl with the ground and fresh ginger, salt, bicarbonate of soda and chocolate chips.

2 Mix together the remaining ingredients, then pour into the bowl and mix well.

3 Form the dough into walnut-sized balls and press down lightly to form little cookies. Transfer to the baking sheet and bake for 12–15 minutes until lightly golden. Leave to cool on the baking sheet for 5 minutes, then transfer to a wire rack to cool completely before serving. (Store in an airtight container for up to 1 week or freeze for 1 month.)

MAKES 12
PREPARATION TIME 10 minutes
COOKING TIME 15 minutes, plus cooling

300g/10½oz/3 cups ground almonds
2 tsp ground ginger
2cm/¾in piece of fresh root ginger, peeled and finely grated
½ tsp sea salt
½ tsp bicarbonate of soda
175g/6oz/1 cup dark chocolate chips
50g/1¾oz/scant ¼ cup almond nut butter or tahini
80g/2¾oz/scant ⅓ cup butter, melted, or melted coconut oil
2¾ tbsp raw honey

NUTRITIONAL INFORMATION PER COOKIE
Protein 6.9g, **Carbohydrates** 14.3g of which sugars 13.5g, **Fat** 27.2g of which saturates 9.7g, **Kcals** 329

HEALTH BENEFITS
The high protein content of these cookies can help to stabilize blood sugar levels, and this too can alleviate sickness. Almonds are a good source of magnesium for healthy nerve function, as well as containing manganese, copper and riboflavin (B2), which are energy-promoting nutrients.

Blueberry Avocado Build-Up Shake

SERVES 2, 250ml/9fl oz/1 cup each
PREPARATION TIME 5 minutes

60g/2¼oz/heaped ⅓ cup blanched almonds
1 tbsp shelled hemp seeds or ground flaxseed
30g/1oz/¼ cup whey vanilla protein powder (optional)
1 ripe avocado, pitted and peeled
150g/5½oz/scant 1 cup fresh or frozen blueberries, plus extra to serve (optional)
300m/10½fl oz/scant 1¼ cups coconut water or water
115ml/3¾fl oz/scant ½ cup coconut milk
115ml/3¾fl oz/scant ½ cup apple juice
2 tsp raw honey or manuka honey (optional)
1 tsp slippery elm powder (optional)
1 tbsp coconut oil (optional)
2 tsp cocoa powder or cacao nibs

Soothing and creamy, thanks to the avocado and coconut milk, this revitalizing berry smoothie is packed with healthy fats, protein, vitamins and minerals. Make it in the morning and sip it throughout the day to help you maintain energy levels.

1 Put the almonds and seeds in a blender or food processor and process until finely ground.

2 Add the remaining ingredients and blend until light and creamy. Serve with more blueberries, if you like. (Store in the fridge for up to 1 day.)

NUTRITIONAL INFORMATION PER SERVING
Protein 8.1g, **Carbohydrates** 31.8g of which sugars 19.9g, **Fat** 26.9g of which saturates 7.3g, **Kcals** 399

HEALTH BENEFITS
Nutrient-dense avocados contain numerous anti-inflammatory compounds including carotenoids, flavonoids, phytosterols, and omega-3 and monounsaturated fats. The phytosterols, which constitute a major proportion of the fats in an avocado, help to lower inflammation. Also included is oleic acid, which helps the body to absorb carotenoids and other fat-soluble nutrients. The unusual mix of anti-inflammatory and antioxidant nutrients found in avocados form the basis of their rich anti-cancer properties.

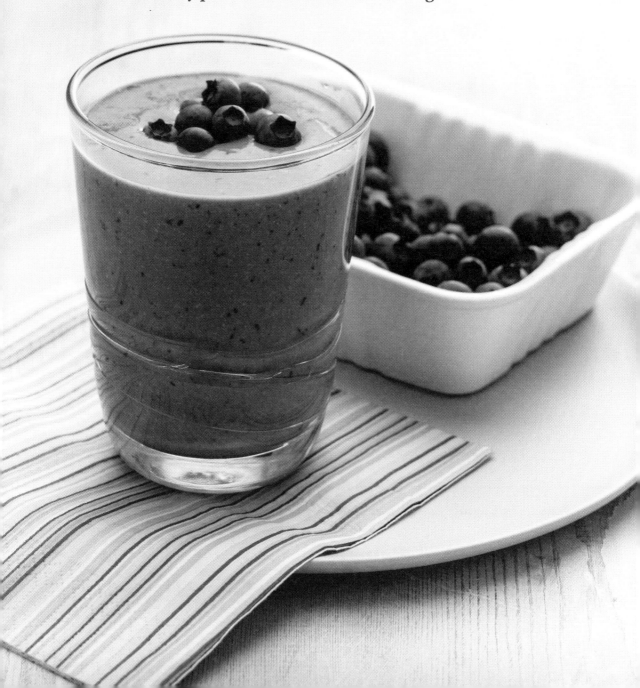

"Shakes and smoothies are ideal during treatment because they provide a nutritious meal in a glass."

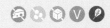

Oat, Almond & Pear Porridge

SERVES 4

PREPARATION TIME 5 minutes

COOKING TIME 10 minutes

200g/7oz/2 cups rolled oats or gluten-free oats

2 ripe pears, cored and chopped

875ml/30fl oz/3½ cups almond or coconut milk

2 tsp cinnamon

80g/2¾oz/¾ cup ground almonds

100ml/3½fl oz/generous ⅓ cup oat cream or coconut cream

2 tbsp ground flaxseed

1½ tbsp chopped or flaked almonds

A warming porridge that is high in protein and healthy fats is a great way to start the day. Ground nuts and seeds provide protein, and the porridge is further enriched with almond milk and oat cream. It makes a strengthening and appealing breakfast to help support your energy levels throughout the morning. The porridge can be made in advance and reheated in the morning with the addition of a little more almond milk.

1 Put the oats, pears, milk and cinnamon into a saucepan. Bring gently to the boil, then lower the heat and simmer for 6–7 minutes, stirring frequently, until the oats are softened and the mixture is thick.

2 Stir in the ground almonds, cream and flaxseed, and beat well. Spoon into bowls and sprinkle the chopped almonds over the porridge to serve.

NUTRITIONAL INFORMATION PER SERVING

Protein 13.9g, **Carbohydrates** 54.4g of which sugars 21.4g, **Fat** 29.9g of which saturates 9.3g, **Kcals** 542

HEALTH BENEFITS

Pears supply natural sweetness while also having a low glycaemic index. They are rich in soluble fibre, which supports blood sugar levels and digestive health. The addition of almonds to this dish provides a useful source of protein and the cancer-protective nutrients manganese and copper. Both of these minerals are important for the production of the key oxidative enzyme superoxide dismutase, which can help protect against damage caused by free radicals.

Cashew & Seed Bars

These raw bars are simple to prepare and provide valuable nutrients as well as protein. Protein helps to support recovery during treatment and to maintain healthy muscle mass, and here it is present in the nuts, seeds and protein powder. The nuts also contain healthy fats and minerals such as copper, manganese, calcium and magnesium.

MAKES 8
PREPARATION TIME 10 minutes,
    plus 1 hour chilling

175g/6oz/scant 1¼ cups cashew nuts
50g/1¾oz/⅓ cup sesame seeds
1 tbsp ground flaxseed
30g/1oz/¼ cup vanilla whey protein
    powder or unsweetened desiccated
    coconut
2 tsp green superfood powder of choice
    (optional)
150g/5½oz/heaped ¾ cup ready-to-eat
    dried apricots
1 tbsp apple juice, if needed

1 Line a baking sheet with baking parchment. Put the nuts into a blender or food processor and process until coarsely ground. Tip into a bowl and add the sesame seeds and flaxseed.

2 Put the protein powder, green superfood powder, if using, and the apricots into a food processor and process to form a sticky dough. Add apple juice, if needed, to bring the mixture together. Add to the nut mixture and mix thoroughly with your hands to form a soft dough.

3 Put the dough on to the prepared baking sheet and use your hands to press it out into a rectangle 2cm/¾in thick. Chill in the fridge for 1 hour to firm up slightly. Cut into 8 bars to serve. (Store in the fridge for up to 1 week or freeze for 1 month.)

NUTRITIONAL INFORMATION PER BAR
Protein 7.7g, **Carbohydrates** 13.4g of which sugars 9.5g, **Fat** 15.6g of which saturates 2.9g, **Kcals** 225

HEALTH BENEFITS
Using the optional green superfood powder, such as spirulina, chlorella or barley grass, is an effective way to increase your intake of nutrients. Being rich in chlorophyll, these powders are particularly alkalizing and potent detoxifiers too.

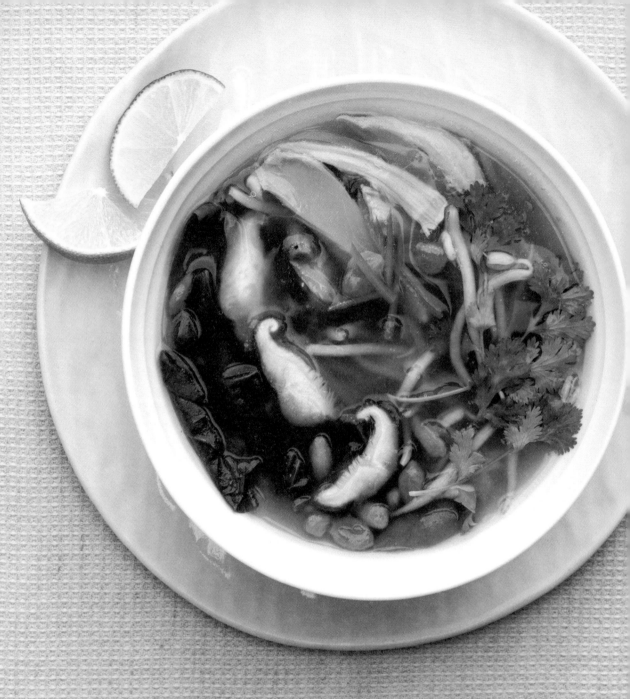

"You can't beat home-made chicken soup
for comfort and healing."

Chicken Ginger Miso Soup

A home-made chicken soup retains all the goodness of the meat and vegetables as well as possessing a pronounced and appetizing flavour. This one includes anti-inflammatory chilli, garlic and ginger, and immune-supporting shiitake mushrooms. The soup can be frozen in batches, making it ideal to prepare during treatment.

1 First make the stock. Put the chicken into a large saucepan and cover with 3l/105fl oz/12 cups water. Add the peppercorns, half the ginger, the onion and 2 garlic cloves, and bring to the boil. Reduce to a simmer and add the fish sauce. Cook for 1 hour or until the meat is tender.

2 Lift out the chicken, then shred the meat. Return the bones to the stock and simmer for 1 hour. Strain the stock and reserve. Discard the vegetables and bones.

3 Boil, then simmer the stock for 10 minutes. Add the remaining ginger and the chicken, spinach, bean sprouts, red onion, chilli, if using, the remaining garlic and the mushrooms. Heat for 2–3 minutes to heat through, then add the goji berries, if using, the lime juice, miso and coriander. Add more fish sauce to taste, if needed. Stir for 1 minute, then serve. (Store in the fridge for up to 3 days or freeze for 1 month.)

SERVES 6
PREPARATION TIME 15 minutes
COOKING TIME 2 hours 20 minutes

1 chicken, 1–1.3kg/2lb 4oz–3lb
1 tsp black peppercorns
6cm/2½in piece of fresh root ginger, peeled and sliced
1 large onion, cut into wedges
4 garlic cloves, crushed
2 tbsp Thai fish sauce, or to taste
1 handful of spinach leaves or 1 pak choi
300g/10½oz/3⅓ cups bean sprouts or sprouted mung beans
1 red onion, finely chopped
1 red chilli, deseeded and finely sliced lengthways (optional)
6 shiitake mushrooms, sliced
3 tbsp goji berries (optional)
a squeeze of lime juice
1 tbsp white sweet miso paste
leaves from 1 bunch of coriander

NUTRITIONAL INFORMATION PER SERVING
Protein 34.7g, **Carbohydrates** 10.2g of which sugars 7.7g, **Fat** 24g of which saturates 6.4g, **Kcals** 396

HEALTH BENEFITS
Chicken is an excellent source of easily digestible protein and of the cancer-protective B vitamin, niacin, as well as selenium. Selenium has been shown to induce DNA repair and synthesis in damaged cells, to inhibit the proliferation of cancer cells and to induce cell death.

SERVES 4
PREPARATION TIME 20 minutes,
    plus 15 minutes soaking
COOKING TIME 30 minutes

12 small shallots, cut in half if large
1 tbsp olive oil
1 tbsp balsamic vinegar
15g/½oz dulse
400g/14oz rice or kelp noodles
12 asparagus spears
1 red pepper, deseeded and cut into
    matchstick strips
8 shiitake mushrooms, sliced
freshly ground black pepper

Dressing
2 tbsp each sesame oil and olive oil
3 tbsp each tamari and balsamic vinegar
a pinch of crushed chillies (optional)
2 tsp raw honey
1 garlic clove, crushed
1cm/½in piece fresh root ginger, peeled
    and grated
1 handful of coriander leaves, chopped

Noodle, Shallot & Shiitake Salad

Rice noodles are perfect for using with a rich balsamic dressing, because they readily absorb the strong flavours. Combined with shiitake mushrooms, asparagus and shallots, they make a satisfying salad. The light-tasting sea vegetable, dulse, is added for its mineral-rich qualities. Just a small handful is sufficient, as it swells once soaked. For protein, add a little cooked flaked salmon or trout.

1   Preheat the oven to 180°C/350°F/Gas 4. Put the shallots in a roasting tin and drizzle with the oil and vinegar. Roast for 30 minutes until golden. Meanwhile, soak the dulse for 15 minutes, then drain and chop.

2   Mix together all the dressing ingredients. Soak the noodles for 3 minutes or according to the packet instructions, then drain and put into a large bowl.

3   Cut the asparagus diagonally into 2cm/¾in pieces, then put it into a steamer and steam over high heat for 1 minute or until just tender. Drain and refresh in cold water. Put the asparagus and shallots into the bowl and add the remaining ingredients. Pour over the dressing and toss to coat. Season with pepper, then serve. (Store, without dressing, in the fridge for up to 3 days.)

NUTRITIONAL INFORMATION PER SERVING
Protein 7g, **Carbohydrates** 73.5g of which sugars 7.1g, **Fat** 11.7g of which saturates 1.7g, **Kcals** 462

HEALTH BENEFITS
Shiitake mushrooms are a powerful immunomodulator, enhancing the function of immune cells in recognizing and destroying cancer cells. Sea vegetables – dulse and the optional kelp noodles – are useful sources of iodine, important in the prevention of breast cancer.

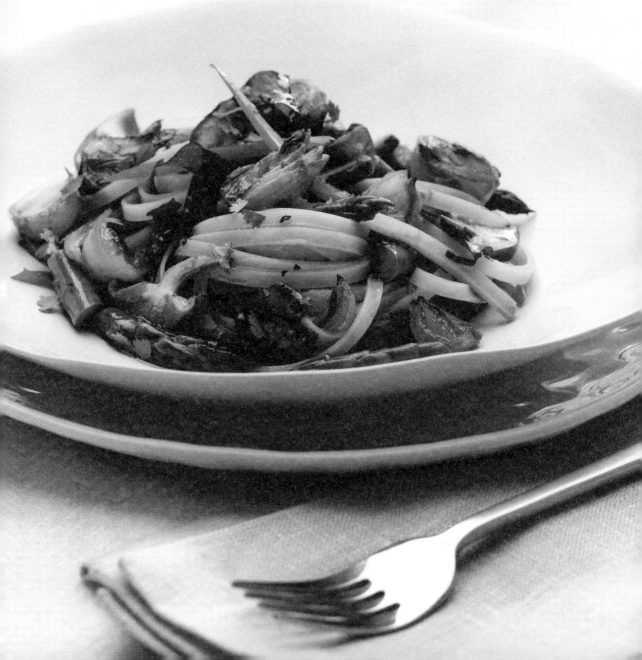

"Benefit from the immune-enhancing properties of sea vegetables and shiitake mushrooms."

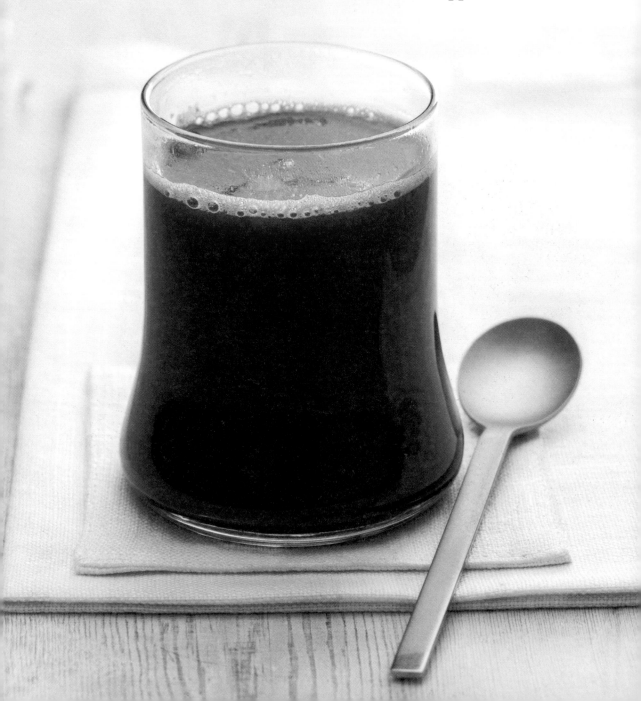

"Relieve flagging energy levels with the benefits of beetroot, cucumber and apple."

Wheatgrass Energizer

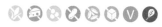

1 Put all the ingredients through an electric juicer. Serve over ice, if you like. Drink immediately.

SERVES 1, 250ml/9fl oz/1 cup
PREPARATION TIME: 5 minutes

1 green apple
1 celery stick
1 handful of spinach
1 bunch of wheatgrass or 1 cube frozen
   wheatgrass
½ lemon
ice cubes, to serve (optional)

NUTRITIONAL INFORMATION PER SERVING
Protein 4.2g, **Carbohydrates** 9.6g of which sugars 9.1g,
Fat 0.6g of which saturates 0.1g, **Kcals** 61

HEALTH BENEFITS
Wheatgrass contains at least 13 vitamins (including antioxidants and B12), minerals and
trace elements, including selenium. It is also a complete source of amino acids (protein
building blocks). Chlorophyll has almost the same molecular structure as haemoglobin
and helps to oxygenate the body.

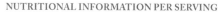

◄ Stamina-Boosting Beetroot Juice

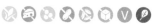

1 Put all the ingredients through an electric juicer. Stir well and drink immediately.

SERVES 1, 250ml/9fl oz/1 cup
PREPARATION TIME 5 minutes

2 apples
1 raw beetroot (about 150g/5½oz)
½ cucumber
½ lemon, peeled

NUTRITIONAL INFORMATION PER SERVING
Protein 4.3g, **Carbohydrates** 27.2g of which sugars 26.9g,
Fat 0.6g of which saturates 0g, **Kcals** 133

HEALTH BENEFITS
Studies have shown that beetroot can increase levels of nitric oxide in the body, which
affects blood flow, hormone levels and cell signalling.

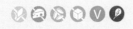

Green Energy Soup

SERVES 4
PREPARATION TIME 10 minutes
COOKING TIME 4 minutes

2 spring onions
½ ripe avocado, pitted and peeled
2 ripe pears, cored
¾ cucumber
1 celery stick
2 tbsp lemon juice
1 tbsp chopped mint leaves, plus extra
   to serve
60g/2¼oz baby spinach leaves or
   watercress
2 tsp ground cumin
a pinch of cayenne pepper
a pinch of sea salt
1 tbsp tamari
250ml/9fl oz/1 cup coconut water, water
   or vegetable stock
freshly ground black pepper
sliced spring onion, to serve

The perfect meal for when you feel too tired to cook: a light, nurturing, super-quick soup that can be served warm or cold. Pears provide natural sweetness to offset the strong flavour of the nutrient-rich spinach. Also included are "hydrating" vegetables – rich in electrolytes, especially potassium – to keep the body's fluids balanced.

1 Put all the ingredients into a blender or food processor and process until smooth. If serving warm, pour the soup into a saucepan and gently warm through for 3–4 minutes, stirring occasionally.
2 Spoon into bowls and serve sprinkled with chopped mint and spring onion, and season with pepper. (Store in the fridge for 1 day.)

NUTRITIONAL INFORMATION PER SERVING
Protein 1.3g, **Carbohydrates** 8.1g of which sugars 8g, **Fat** 2.9g of which saturates 0.5g, **Kcals** 63

HEALTH BENEFITS
Spinach is a rich source of folate and also contains vitamin B6. Folate, plus B6 and methionine, can help the body to protect and repair DNA, and therefore these nutrients play an important role in inhibiting cancer development. B vitamins are also needed for energy production. Also contained are phytonutrients and some unique anti-cancer carotenoids, called epoxyxanthophylls.

Chicken Liver Salad with Cider Vinegar Dressing

Nutrient-rich greens contrast with sweet apple and crunchy walnuts in this salad to serve with chicken livers – brought together with a tangy dressing. Choose organic liver, if you can, as it provides the greatest health benefits.

1 Lightly toast the walnuts in a dry frying pan over medium heat for 1 minute, stirring, then chop them roughly. Set aside. Remove the sinew from the livers, and cut the livers in half if large. Season with salt and pepper and set aside.

2 Tear the lettuce and watercress and put it into a bowl with the apple, celery and parsley. Whisk the dressing ingredients together and season. Spoon 1–2 tablespoons over the leaves and toss to lightly coat. Add the walnuts and toss lightly. Divide on to four plates.

3 Heat the olive oil in a large, heavy-based frying pan over medium heat. Fry the livers for 3–4 minutes on each side until golden brown and just cooked through to the centre. Remove from the heat and arrange on the salad leaves.

4 Put the remaining dressing in the pan. Allow it to bubble for a few seconds, then drizzle over the salad and serve. (Store, without dressing, in the fridge for up to 1 day.)

SERVES 4
PREPARATION TIME 10 minutes
COOKING TIME 10 minutes

100g/3½oz/heaped ¾ cup walnut pieces
   or pecan nuts
400g/14oz chicken livers
1 large head of romaine lettuce or other
   lettuce
2 small handfuls of watercress
1 apple, diced
2 celery sticks, finely diced
2 tbsp chopped parsley leaves
1 tbsp olive oil, ghee or coconut oil
sea salt and freshly ground black pepper

Cider vinegar dressing
2 tbsp apple cider vinegar
1 tsp Dijon mustard
5 tbsp olive oil

NUTRITIONAL INFORMATION PER SERVING
Protein 22.9g, **Carbohydrates** 4.5g of which sugars 4.4g, **Fat** 33.6g of which saturates 6.3g, **Kcals** 412

HEALTH BENEFITS
Chicken liver is an exceptionally nutrient-dense food, an excellent source of zinc, vitamins B12 and A, copper, selenium and protein, and a good source of iron – especially important for relieving fatigue and energizing the body.

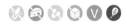

Coconut Cocoa Booster

SERVES 2
PREPARATION TIME 5 minutes

2 tsp cocoa powder or raw cacao powder,
    or to taste
1 tsp maca powder
1 tbsp ground flaxseed
250ml/9fl oz/1 cup coconut milk
250ml/9fl oz/1 cup coconut water or
    water
2 tsp coconut oil (optional)
1 banana
2 tbsp seeds or nuts, to serve

1 Put all the ingredients into a blender or food processor and process until smooth. Drink immediately or store in the fridge for up to 1 day. To serve hot, heat the blended drink gently in a saucepan until hot but not boiling. Serve each drink with 1 tablespoon seeds or nuts.

NUTRITIONAL INFORMATION PER SERVING
Protein 4.5g, **Carbohydrates** 28g of which sugars 16g,
Fat 7.3g of which saturates 3.4g, **Kcals** 194

HEALTH BENEFITS
Maca is a Peruvian root that can be bought in powdered form. It has been used traditionally to support the body in times of stress. (Maca can also be used in baking.)

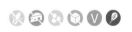

Chia Papaya Pudding ▸

SERVES 2
PREPARATION TIME 5 minutes,
    plus 15 minutes soaking

4 tbsp chia seeds
6 pitted dried dates
90g/3¼oz/scant ⅔ cup cashew nuts
a pinch of cinnamon
a pinch of sea salt
1 ripe papaya, peeled, deseeded and
    sliced
2 tbsp flaked coconut

1 Soak the chia seeds in water for 15 minutes. Put all the ingredients, except the papaya and coconut, into a blender or food processor with 500ml/17fl oz/2 cups water and process until smooth. Serve topped with the papaya and coconut. (Store in the fridge for up to 1 day.)

NUTRITIONAL INFORMATION PER SERVING
Protein 7.5g, **Carbohydrates** 18.1g of which sugars 6.3g,
Fat 20.2g of which saturates 6.6g, **Kcals** 281

HEALTH BENEFITS
Chia seeds are rich in omega-3 and easily digestible protein and fibre. Papaya contains protective antioxidants and the digestive enzyme, papain.

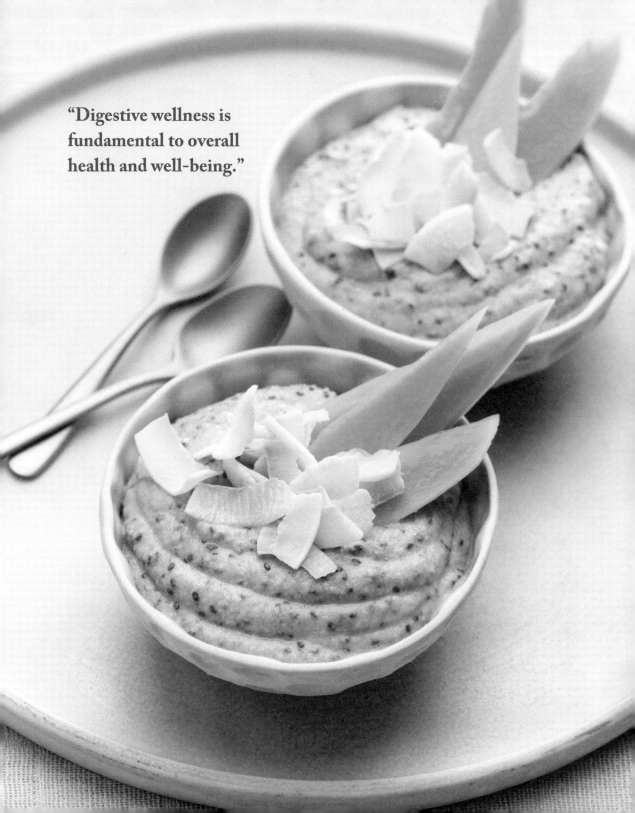

"Digestive wellness is fundamental to overall health and well-being."

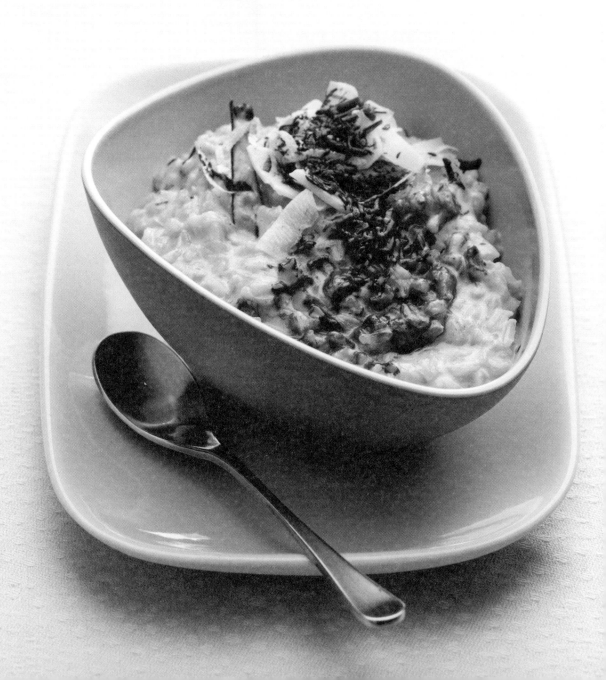

"Richly flavoured yet beautifully soothing for the digestion."

Coconut Rice Pudding

Toasting the rice in the butter gives it a lovely nuttiness, which is complemented by the caramel flavour of the molasses. Adding a dash of molasses gives sweetness to the dessert as well as providing potassium, calcium and iron. B vitamins, soluble fibre and slow-releasing complex carbohydrate are also present.

1 Heat the butter in a large pan over medium heat and add the rice. Stir to coat in the butter for 2–3 minutes to create a nutty flavour.
2 Pour in the coconut milk, vanilla extract, cinnamon stick, and lemon zest and juice. Bring to the boil, then lower the heat and simmer for 30 minutes, stirring occasionally.
3 Add the molasses, flaxseed, coconut flakes and most of the chocolate, and cook for a further 10–15 minutes, stirring occasionally. The rice should be very tender and most of the liquid should be absorbed. Remove the pan from the heat and leave the rice to stand, covered, for 5 minutes. Serve warm or chilled, and sprinkle the remaining chocolate on top with a few coconut flakes and lemon zest, if you like. (You can add all the chocolate at the beginning of step 3 if you prefer.) (Store in the fridge for up to 2 days.)

SERVES 6
PREPARATION TIME 5 minutes
COOKING TIME 50 minutes,
   plus 5 minutes standing

2 tbsp butter or coconut oil
350g/12oz/1⅔ cups long grain brown rice
1.25l/44fl oz/5 cups coconut milk
1 tsp vanilla extract
1 cinnamon stick, broken in half
zest and juice of 1 lemon, plus extra zest
   to serve (optional)
1 tbsp molasses
1 tbsp ground flaxseed
30g/1oz/½ cup coconut flakes, plus extra
   to serve (optional)
20g/¾oz dark chocolate (at least 75%
   cocoa solids), grated, or 1 tbsp cacao
   nibs

NUTRITIONAL INFORMATION PER SERVING
Protein 5.4g, **Carbohydrates** 57.7g of which sugars 13.8g, **Fat** 9.9g of which saturates 6.5g, **Kcals** 342

HEALTH BENEFITS
The soluble fibre in the rice is gentle on the digestive system and useful for relieving diarrhoea and constipation. Coconut milk and coconut oil provide a source of lauric acid for immune health and caprylic acid to support the gut.

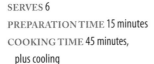

Italian Crackers & Bean Dip

SERVES 6

PREPARATION TIME 15 minutes

COOKING TIME 45 minutes, plus cooling

250g/9oz/1½ cups flaxseeds

50g/1¾oz/⅓ cup almonds

1 red pepper, deseeded and chopped

1 tomato, chopped

1 egg

zest and juice of ½ lemon

60g/2¼oz/½ cup pitted black olives

1 tbsp chopped basil leaves

sea salt and freshly ground black pepper

Curried bean dip

400g/14oz/2 cups tinned cannellini beans, drained and rinsed

1 tsp turmeric

2 garlic cloves

½ tsp ground cumin

1 tbsp lemon juice

about 2 tbsp olive oil

1 tbsp chopped parsley leaves

Baking these crackers in a low oven preserves their omega-3 content. Serve them as a snack or for a light meal with the dip, which contains cancer-protective turmeric.

1 Preheat the oven to 150°C/300°F/Gas 2 and line a baking sheet with baking parchment. Grind the flaxseeds and almonds in a food processor until fine. Add the red pepper and tomato, and process until combined.

2 Add the egg, lemon zest and juice, then season with salt and pepper. Process to form a thick dough. Briefly pulse in the black olives and stir in the basil.

3 Using a spatula and damp hands, spread the mixture onto the baking sheet to 5mm/¼in thick, then shape into a square. Score lines to make individual crackers. Bake for 40–45 minutes until golden and crisp.

4 Put all the ingredients for the curried bean dip into a food processor and season lightly. Process until smooth. Add a little extra oil if needed.

5 Break the flaxseed mixture into individual crackers along the score lines and leave to cool on a wire rack. Serve with the dip. (Store the crackers in an airtight container for up to 4 days. Store the dip in the fridge for up to 3 days.)

NUTRITIONAL INFORMATION PER SERVING OF CRACKERS

Protein 3.3g, **Carbohydrates** 4.4g of which sugars 1.1g, **Fat** 7.6g of which saturates 0.8g, **Kcals** 95

NUTRITIONAL INFORMATION PER SERVING OF DIP

Protein 2.4g, **Carbohydrates** 4.7g of which sugars 0.5g, **Fat** 3.3g of which saturates 0.5g, **Kcals** 57

HEALTH BENEFITS

The fibre content helps support overall digestive health, which is particularly important in reducing the risk of bowel cancer.

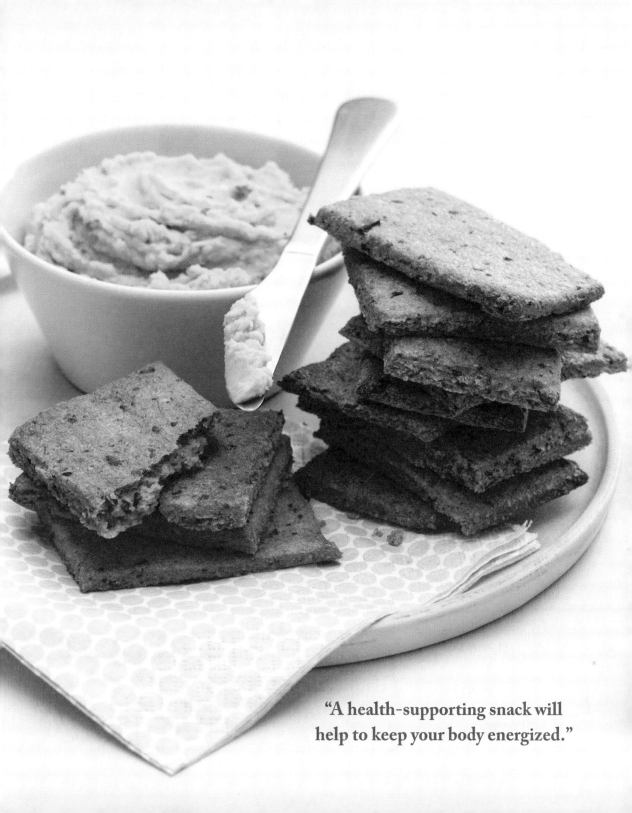

"A health-supporting snack will
help to keep your body energized."

Index